OWL HILL

By: Harold Hinson

authorHOUSE®

AuthorHouse™
1663 Liberty Drive
Bloomington, IN 47403
www.authorhouse.com
Phone: 1-800-839-8640

First published by AuthorHouse 9/22/2009

ISBN: 978-1-4490-1727-9 (e)
ISBN: 978-1-4490-1725-5 (sc)
ISBN: 978-1-4490-1726-2 (hc)

Library of Congress Control Number: 2009909435

Printed in the United States of America
Bloomington, Indiana

This book is printed on acid-free paper.

DEDICATION PAGE

Dedicated to my wife, Faye,
and our two sons,
Todd and Scott

"The grace of our Lord Jesus Christ be with you all." Amen.

Revelation 22:21
Holy Bible, King James Version

TABLE OF CONTENTS

INTRODUCTION

Owl Hill is a true story about a man born into deep poverty, raised by his devout religious mother and his alcoholic father. Married at the age of 17, served four years active duty in the United States Air Force, successfully employed in the corporate industry for 40 years. With his wife raised two Christian young men that became leaders in their respective churches. His life gets exposed to relatives being murdered, relatives committing suicide, and dramatic career changes in midlife. His wife suffers severe pain on numerous occasions partially due to negligent surgical procedures that ultimately leads to her loss of memory and then to her diagnosis of Alzheimer's/dementia. This man spends his 55th wedding anniversary with his wife as her caretaker and explains in detail how Alzheimer's/dementia began, and continues to affect their lives.

Chapter I
My Beginning

It was April 1936 and spring was in the air. At 430PM, my dad walked up Owl Hill's old rocky dirt road after getting off work at Chatham Manufacturing Company and entered the old frame house with a tin roof he rented from Chatham's for $4.32 per month. He grabbed my mom's hand and led her upstairs, laid her down on the floor between the two beds on a hand-braided rug she had made from salvage and together they made a baby.

Nine months later on January 29, 1937, I was born, Shelly Harold Hinson, delivered by our old family doctor, Dr. Samuel Gambill. That is the story my mom told me after I became an adult and I have no reason not to believe her. She was 24 but she was only 15 when they were married and their first child was born eight years earlier, when she was 16, so I guess my dad decided time was wasting. He wanted another baby and he wanted it now. Dr. Gambill was our family doctor who in this time period made house calls. If you wanted to visit the doctor, you went to his house. He had no office other than his house as was the case with most doctors in Elkin, North Carolina. He also had the "medicine" he would prescribe so you didn't have to go to a drug store with a prescription as you would today. It may be snake oil or heavy on alcohol, though.

My dad was born Winfield Shelly Hinson in Wilkes County on

February 28, 1899. His family owned and operated a farm. He had a twin brother named Dewey and when they were old enough to leave home, they did just that. I can barely remember my Grandpa Charlie Columbus Hinson. He weighed 300 pounds and had lost a leg after stepping on a rusty nail and taking gangrene. He would spend his days sitting in a chair in the doorway to the porch looking out over his farmland. He died November 19, 1942, when I was only 5 years old. His condition meant the five boys he and Grandma Nancy had would be responsible for working the farm. Farm life for my dad just was not what he and Dewey wanted to do. So, somehow in their teens they migrated to Winston-Salem and landed work with the famous wagon manufacturer, Nissen Wagon Works, located in the Waughtown section of Winston-Salem. They made enough money to partner an old T-Model together and were living in a boarding house where they could eat and sleep for one price. This was what they had dreamed about and here they were living their dream.

Their dream diminished, though, when Dewey came down with pneumonia and it was back to the farm for both of them. One could not leave without the other.

My dad then took a job with the WPA and helped build the dirt road from Wilkes County to the top of the Blue Ridge Mountain. The only equipment they had were the mules and drag pans to move the dirt. It was a back breaking job and that ended pretty soon too.

So, it was back to more working on the farm.

Determined not to have to work on the farm, no pay and no respect, dad went to Chatham Manufacturing Company and was hired to work in the dye house. That is where they dyed the warp and wool that they used to make blankets and automobile upholstery.

Automobile upholstery was a big market for Chatham's and their blankets were known worldwide. Dad now had no transportation. Dewey kept the T-Model so he had to live in another boarding house since the farm was too far to walk to and from his new job. My dad never had a driver's license or owned an automobile from that day forward.

This is about the time he met my mom. She was born Opal Ophelia Gentry on May 31, 1912, and was also raised on a farm in an area called Friendship Community. The Gentry family owned probably several hundred acres or more and my Grandpa Decatur Gentry was also a farmer but he owned and operated a sawmill and was a very popular source for corn liquor.

That's white lightning, the race car driver Junior Johnson made it famous in later years. Matter of fact, grandpa spent time in Atlanta Penitentiary about the same time Al Capone was a resident at the same facility. That was sometime around 1932.

Mom wrote about her and dad first meeting. She said it was on a Saturday night at an entertainment of fiddle and banjo picking at the Cambric School House. The place was packed. Papa, the name she used for grandpa, momma, her step mom, Omar, her brother, and Mae Collins were there. Mom's real mother died when she was nine years old. He was actually married five times and his wives are buried beside him in a single row at the Friendship Baptist Church Cemetery.

Mom and Ruby, who was mom's sister, and a lot of other people were just standing against the wall along the big high long porch outside.

Shelly came up the steps wearing a gray, tweed suit and gray hat with a wide dark band on it. Mom had on a mingled gray coat she said with a gray fur collar and a wide linen, dark green velvet hat with a light green silk lining under the brim. She was only fifteen.

A man named Bonson Layell came to her at least three times and asked if he could take her home. He was drinking, or just couldn't be still, and she told him she didn't know him and to let her alone.

Shelly stepped up to her and said, if you don't want to have any thing to do with him, I'll slap the "sol" out of him, and stood there by her the rest of the evening. Never knew what "sol" was. Then he asked if he could take her home. Mom said I don't know you either.

He told her his name which she forgot, except Hinson. He said, you stay right here till I go to the house and get my car, which was actually his and his twin brother Dewey's. I walked up here, he said.

Just as he drove up in his T-Model, papa and all of us were driving away. Mom said she told papa a man wanted to take me home. He said, who? I forgot his name she said so papa told her to come on and go with us. I was sorry I left and I worried about it, mom says.

Mr. T. C. Deborde, who rode a horse to teach school, spent the night at mom's house when it rained. Papa boarded all the teachers at our house anyway for $18.00 a month. This was in 1926-1927.

Mom says one night when Mr. DeBorde stayed with them, momma told me to ask him if he knew any Hinson's up his way. He said he did, one hauls wood by his house on Bridge Street and one worked at Chatham's. That is all he knew. She asked if they were married and he said one was.

Well, mom said she was going to school and she knew where most of the others lived about so she decided to get up and go sit with

Tina Cave. She was later the widow of Walt Dula, descendants of the legendary Tom Dula, sometimes pronounced Dooley. According to Wikipedia Tom Dula was from the Appalachia hill country in Wilkes County, North Carolina. He was the youngest of three brothers. He was convicted of the murder of his lover Laura Foster who disappeared May 25, 1866. Tom Dula was hanged in 1868 in Statesville, North Carolina. The Kingston Trio made him a legend with the ballad "Hang Down Your Head Tom Dooley." Now, we were all young mom said, but she just had to find Shelly. She felt bad about leaving him and she liked the looks of him.

Tina told her a Hinson went around with her uncle Ted White. She said his name was Shelly. Then she remembered, that was the name he told her at the entertainment that night at Cambric School.

Weeks passed and April Fools Day came. We wrote silly little verses mom said, signed guess who and passed them around at school. So, she told Tina she was going to mail one and Tina helped her that April Fools Day. She mailed, I saw you at Cambric. I go to school at Rock Springs. I live in a great big house with a great big cherry tree and a well in front. Guess who?

More time passed and finally he found her, she said. He said, here you are, a friend of mine Ted White told me Gentry's live down here. I've been down here once before looking for you. The yard was full of girls and boys playing games.

He had gotten the silly little verse she had written and came to see her every other Sunday for a while after that.

One Sunday mom said, he swept me off my feet. He asked me if she had a regular fellow. She told him no, I go with all of them, any one that asked to walk me from church which was a mile and crowds of us. He said, well you have now. I've decided that I'm not going to see Bea Spicer any more, I want to come see you.

This was the first of June and he never missed a Saturday night or a Sunday for the next three months. When she asked him to come back on Wednesday nights because it was so long from Sunday to Saturday he said he couldn't, he had to work.

You see, he had already been working at Chatham's for five years.

So one thing led to another really fast and they were married September 3, 1927. He was 28, she was only 15.

There was not much interaction between me and my older brother Charlie. He was eight years old when I was born, so by the time he was 16 and going out with the girls, I was just finding out the difference between boys and girls. Charlie made a positive difference in my life, though, which I will always cherish forever. First of all, he bought my first "new" bicycle that my parents probably could not afford. He helped build my parent's second home place with labor and financial aid. He carried me home with him for a visit when he was in the Air Force and stationed at Marysville, Tennessee. That was the first time I had ever been away from home. His wife, Nell Johnson from Taylorsville, North Carolina, made us a banana pudding since she knew I loved banana pudding. When the bowl was handed to me, it slipped out of my hands and dropped onto the table shattering the bowl and splattering the banana pudding all over everything. I was so embarrassed I cried. He arranged my first job selling popcorn and soft drinks at the Valley Drive Inn Theater, which he helped managed. That led me to getting the position of projectionist when Bud Durham, who was the projectionist, died in a car accident. I drove his 1951 blue and white Ford hardtop with white leather seats on my first major date at 16. He provided financial assistance to our parents when they needed it most and I could not afford to do so.

Charlie made it possible for us to drive his just purchased Lincoln from North Carolina to Alaska to visit him and while in Alaska, arranged and paid for a cruise through Prince William Sound via Portage Glacier and other glaciers for my family of four. It was the thrill of a lifetime.

When Charlie fell ill to cancer he was transferred from Alaska where he lived to San Francisco for surgery. I managed to go visit with him and his wife during his surgery in California.

Then, when his condition further deteriorated I was able to travel to Alaska and was with him when he passed away. It was the very least I could have done for my older brother.

Charlie was a very motivated individual. He usually held two jobs at once and sometimes three. He told me on occasions that if he didn't have to sleep he could make some real money. I guess his first job was stoking the furnace for Louis Mitchell's apartments and that position also provided him a room since the coal fired furnace had to be fed day and night to keep the building and its tenants warm. While he was doing that he was also dispatching cabs for the local cab company there in Elkin. But if that wasn't enough, he was also a short order cook for the Eat Quick Cafe. When he went to work for Chatham Manufacturing Company, though, he had to slow down to maybe just two jobs because that was an 8 hour day job and he worked midnight shift for a while.

He always complained he didn't have time to sleep.

Charlie spent in excess of twenty years in the United States Air Force. It was strange, though, he never went across the Atlantic or Pacific. His tours of duty consisted of Canada, Newfoundland, and, of course, Alaska. This is where he settled after retiring from the Air Force.

In Alaska, his work schedule was same as before, when he was off duty it was to another job. One of those was a trucking company that moved containers off and on ships. Another job was owner of a truck distributor of natural gas. He also owned and rented apartments and a host of other things to keep him busy and bringing in the cash.

When the Air Force transferred him to Alaska, he was living in a mobile home. Knowing how expensive it would be living in Alaska, he made arrangements to have that mobile home towed to Alaska and that was when the ALCAN Highway was about one thousand miles of dirt and gravel unpaved road. I forget how many flat tires the towing company had on the trailer but when it arrived after traveling one thousand miles on a gravel dirt road, everything inside that was glass was destroyed, including the commodes. If it wasn't destroyed, it was shook loose from where it was. In addition to the breakage, there was a couple inches of dust and dirt that had also filtered inside. It was a mess to be cleaned up, for sure.

When I turned three, my dad apparently took mom back upstairs and laid her down on that braided rug again that she had made years earlier and, you guessed it, they made another baby. Samuel, (Sam) my little brother, was born in 1941 and again, he was also delivered by Dr. Samuel Gambill.. He was also given his namesake, Samuel. The day all this was to happen they decided I shouldn't be around for the occurrence so I was taken to one of our neighbors to play.

One of the kids my age was also at the Walker's house. His name was Clarence Swaim.

On the previous Christmas, Santa Claus had brought me a really sharp Radio Flyer wooden wagon with wood sideboards. I rode in that wagon up the old rocky dirt road to the Walker's house which was about three or four houses away and they placed it up on the front porch for us to play in. The porch was about three to four feet off the ground and had no rails or banisters to protect us from falling off.

Lo and behold, Clarence gave that wagon a big shove and it went sailing off the porch landing on the ground with the tongue and front wheels first, ripping the front wheels from the wooden bed in what we would call today a total wreck.

Fortunately, neither of us was in the wagon at the time but that was the worst day of my life at three years old. I cried and cried and cried some more. This is one of those things that gets burned into your brain and you seem to never forget.

Sam and I were pretty close from the very beginning. When he graduated from the crib, he and I slept upstairs in the same bed across from Charlie's bed with the famous braided rug on the floor between the two beds. Sometimes when we went to bed we would hum out loud when Charlie was at work until our hums harmonized. We would hold our breath and do it over and over again. Then when dad tapped on the wall in the bedroom down below, we knew it was time to knock it off.

We played about as hard as you possibly could with the toy cars and trucks. I bet we hauled enough dirt in those toy trucks to fill a real dump truck. In our front yard was a really big oak tree and its roots were exposed running out in the yard. No grass would ever grow under that old oak and we made sure of it by keeping the dirt moving. Between our house and the house next door was what we called a holler. It was about one hundred feet wide and probably fifty feet deep and tapered off back into the woods behind the houses.

Chatham's operated a sawmill on site and they began hauling the sawdust up Owl Hill Road and started filling in the deep holler. Now talking about a playground, we had one super place to play. Never got muddy, never stayed wet, and was right next door. After a while when you would dig down into the sawdust it would get warm and the further you dug the warmer it got. They told us it was on fire deep inside. Next to the road where they were dumping this sawdust was a beechnut tree. The branches of it hung out over the road and we would climb the tree and sit on a limb and watch the cars go past directly underneath of us. We would also eat the nuts but they were awfully bitter, especially when they were still green.. My initials and many others were carved all over the trunk of that beechnut tree.

Charlie bought brand new bicycles for me and Sam one Christmas so we retired the old clunkers we kept repairing with parts from Mr. Elmore's Store located downtown in Elkin. These actually had fenders, a horn, a light, chain guard, and the works. Prior to that, though, if we could find enough wheels, Sam and I could make a ride. Sam had no fear. As a teenager he could remove a transmission from his car, he could rebuild a carburetor, he drove a dragster in competition and ventured out west and worked in the wheat/corn fields for one season.

I didn't have Sam's talent but together he and I would tackle about any project, from remodeling a house to building sun decks.

Together we could do it all.

We lost Sam in a single automobile accident and it was never the same. During our early marriages, we traveled to many places together, from the beach to the mountains, to Nashville to Cincinnati. We even purchased identical cars in 1979, Dodge Magnums, same color and same style. They had unique grills and when we parked in motel parking lots we would back in so the two grills would be sitting side by side. I still miss Sam.

Chapter 2
Owl Hill Community

From Highway 268 at the Chatham entrance to the old Hugh Chatham Hospital was a crooked, rocky, dirt road that took you through Owl Hill. This area was owned by Chatham's and consisted of about 14 company owned houses. At least one resident of each house was employed by Chatham's to qualify for their subsidized rent. Each house had plenty of space for a garden or whatever and was not crammed together at all. We actually had a cow, a mule, hogs, and a garden. The mule was kind of a community mule. It was shared among those that wanted to plant a garden and could handle a mule. The cow grazed the back side all the way to the woods and the hog pen was in between.

Now these houses were not elaborate by any means of the imagination. There was no running hot water, no indoor toilet, no heating system or, heaven forbids, air condition. Your hot water came from the kitchen stove that had a water jacket attached. Your indoor toilet consisted of a chamber maid (slop jar), and the heat was from either a fireplace or a wood burning stove.

The daytime toilet was down a path between the hog pen and the garden with an never ending supply of paper, the Sears Roebuck catalog.

Sometimes our old cow would eat wild onions and that would

make the milk taste like wild onions. Then occasionally the milk would spoil when the block of ice from Ipock Coal and Ice would melt before our next delivery of ice was made. In addition to that, milk at school was supplied by Klondike Farms and served in glass bottles. It had about an inch of cream on top and if you didn't shake it up real good, it was really nasty. So, I got turned against milk at an early age and I don't much care for it to this day.

Since we knew we would have to empty the chamber maid the next morning, Sam and I decided we would open the window and urinate through the screen which would run down on the tin roof over the front porch and on the ground. That was cool except after a while the urine rusted the screen wire and caused it to rot and the stream running down the tin roof started to stain a bright brown rust color on the tin.

All the houses on Owl Hill were wood frame, German siding, wood beaded ceilings, linoleum on the floors. There was no underpinning and no insulation, no carpets. They were hard to heat, but Ipock delivered the coal for our fireplace and ice for our ice box.

On really cold nights, Sam and I would get the pillow from our bed and warm it in front of the fireplace and then run upstairs and jump in bed and wrap up with the warmed pillow. Never knew any time that we were cold or deprived of heat as a result of this system.

In the winter we would kill hogs and that was a community effort as well. My dad always raised two hogs each year and killing time was after Thanksgiving when the temperature was cold enough so the meat would not spoil. A large vat was placed over a good hot fire and then the hog was either shot in the head or hit in the head with a hammer. It was then placed in the hot boiling water and all the hair was scrapped from the hide. After the hog's skin was clean from all its hair, it was hung up on a scaffold-like apparatus by its hind legs. There it was cut open and all the intestines removed. We didn't throw much away either. Mom made liver mush (liver pudding) from the liver, chitlins from the intestines, and lard from the grease that cooked out. The head (jowls) made good fatback for frying and seasoning. The hind quarters were salt preserved to become country ham and the front quarters were used for sausage along with some of the side meat. The other side meat was our bacon. Our smokehouse was the primary storage for the meat after it was salt preserved and we had meat year around. My dad loved pork but he really didn't like beef. He could work all day with scalding a hog and scraping and cutting it up and the odor didn't bother him one bit. But killing a cow and doing the same thing had such an odor to him it would make him nearly vomit. You might say we never had beef on our table when I was growing up. None.

When our corn that was saved to feed the hogs dried out in the fall, we would shell it and save the cobs. The corn was taken to Carter's Mill, a local mill, and had it ground into feed. That way you didn't have to buy so much to feed the hogs and the feed was placed in pretty floral sacks. Mom made skirts out of feed sacks for herself and some were actually pieced together to make bed sheets. The cobs were put in a box and placed inside the outdoor toilet. These were our alternate tissue when the Sears Roebuck catalog pages started to run out. Our outhouse was a two-seater but I never knew any two people to use it at the same time.

Most of our vegetables were grown in the garden, corn, beans, squash, tomatoes, limas, cabbage, and lettuce, among others. Mom would can what she could to preserve them for the winter. Our ice box with a block of ice wouldn't do much for freezing so that was out of the question. The Mason jars were washed and stored for the next season as we used up what we needed for the table.

The groceries that we didn't have such as flour, sugar and regular staples came from W. W. Whitaker's store. Mom would make a list of what she needed and on Saturday when we went to town, drop it off and he would pick the items and deliver them to our house.

He would back into the driveway to the back door and take them in the house and put them on the kitchen table whether we were home or not. There would always be a bag of candy in the groceries and Sam and I would divide it between us. Sometimes if it was a candy bar I would try to divide it so that my half was the biggest. It didn't work very often. We always went to town on Saturday. Sometimes we would walk, sometimes we would get a ride from a neighbor. Mom and Dad would take Sam and me to the motion picture theater and leave us. Dad would go to the barber shop and get his weekly shower. Mom would "shop." Then when the show was over they would meet us at the theater and we would go back home. Sometimes my dad would stop by the pool room and partake of the juices they served there and sometimes it was more than he should have partaken. But he was known for that all along. At home he kept hidden a quart or half gallon of corn liquor (white lightning) and somehow he would start showing his indulgence and we hadn't seen him take a drink.

Speaking of sipping the juice, we had one rowdy dude on Owl Hill that was known to drink a little too much and he was in his late teens. He was old enough to drive and owned a 1936 Ford that knew how to take the dirt road curves with a controlled slide.

When he was in this condition, going around the curves the gravel would be thrown almost to your front door. You could always hear him coming up the road from the sound of the gravel.

One day he took one of the curves right below our house just a little too fast and he turned that old '36 Ford over on its side. Everybody that saw it just knew old rowdy had killed himself.

By the time we all got to where it was laying on its side, old rowdy climbed out the passenger side window and was smiling from ear to ear. He was in fact about 3 sheets in the wind. Staggering around to see what condition he was in he summoned some of the adult bystanders to help him roll it back on its wheels. Sure enough, they were able to do just that. Once back on the four wheels, old rowdy got back in, started it up and drove on his way. Old rowdy lived to challenge death one more time.

Roy Chipman was our next door neighbor with the sawdust playground between us. He and his wife, Ethel, had three girls and one boy, Jim, Mary Sue, Wilma, and Dot. Also living in the Chipman house was Sonny Blackburn, Cooper McBride, and Polly Chipman. Cooper was Ethel's sister and Sonny and Polly were first cousins. Never knew why these people were part of the Chipman household. The Chipman's had a buffet that she stored leftovers and a Kelvinator refrigerator that had a motor on the top of the unit in a big round ball.

We didn't have a buffet or a refrigerator but we did have an ice box.

Roy's family had the first telephone that I knew of on Owl Hill. It was a "party line" which means there are about eight other people on the same line and you have to wait if someone else is on the line when you pickup. You can hear their conversation and they can tell when you picked up by a click in their receiver. When you wanted to make a call, you picked up the handset and an operator would answer immediately by saying "number please." You gave the operator the number you wanted to call like City Cabs, for instance, I remember their number was 292. The operator connected you to number 292 and City Cabs would answer. I remember this number because sometimes we were allowed to use their telephone to call a cab when it was raining and we needed to go out or call a friend or relative for various reasons.

We didn't have a telephone the entire time we lived on Owl Hill and not many of our neighbors had one either.

The Chipman's also had the first electric lawn mower I had ever seen. We didn't have enough grass for a lawn mower at our house. If the grass between the pig pen and the outhouse got tall enough my dad would use an old sling blade to knock it down. This electric lawn mower was really neat, though. The motor was real quiet and you could hardly hear it running. The problems I saw with it, however, the motor was not strong enough to mow any reasonable tall grass without choking down. Sometimes when that happened it would blow a fuse. The second problem was keeping the electric cord out of the way of the blade. I witnessed that problem one day when the person mowing ran over the cord and severed it. Electric sparks flew and a spliced extension cord was necessary to continue.

Roy was a carpenter by trade and a supervisor at Chatham's. He was instrumental in building the Camp Butler campground where young people could go during the school summer break. The construction took place near Sparta, North Carolina, at the top of the Blue Ridge Mountains and occasionally he would come home with some type of wild animal they had captured during the construction just to show it to the neighborhood because most of us had never seen such animals. One of these animals was a raccoon. He put a collar on it like a puppy dog and led it around the neighborhood for all the kids to see.

Another time he brought home a skunk. He said they had deodorized it but you couldn't prove it by me 'cause it still smelled pretty bad.

Roy was another one that liked the juice. Often he would be at our house looking at the hogs or just a casual meeting for a nip.

Funny thing, he always had a pocket full of change. After he had a nip or two he would gather all the kids in sight and take that pocket full of change and toss it up in the air as high as he could just to watch the kids scramble to see who could find the most money. We as kids looked forward to it but in hind site, it was his entertainment. The money I picked up went into my piggy bank. It was one that had no opening to get the money out and you could barely squeeze a dime out by shaking it upside down. When it was full, you took a hammer to it and went to the store to buy candy or a toy.

We often visited the Chipman's on Friday or Saturday nights for a game of rook. They all really liked to play cards. There was no gambling but the skill of bidding and making your bid was as challenging as it gets. After one game of 300 points, they would usually switch partners and let someone else in on the game of four people so that everybody that wanted to play would get a chance. Sometimes they would let Wilma and me play after their juice started affected their playing. Roy would sometimes call Wilma a tomboy and that didn't set well with me. I thought Wilma was really pretty and no way like a tomboy. I actually had a crush on her and tried to express my feelings but she never showed me any in return.

Approaching midnight, Ethel would fix a big pot of oyster stew and the games would end with a bowl. I didn't like stewed oysters so I always picked mine out and just ate the soup. It was good. She also served little round oyster crackers with the soup. At our house we didn't have oyster crackers, we just used regular old saltine crackers. They were cheaper and we used them for multiple purposes like with a slice of cheese.

Roy was a talented man and he helped build my parent's second house in 1949 when Chatham's asked everybody to move so they could expand.

Mom's sister, Ruby, lived just up the road a few houses and she worked at Chatham's. I can't recall her husband, Aubrey, ever having a job at public work. Also, I can't recall him ever being sober. My dad didn't have much to do with him because of the differences in them.

My dad did his nipping on Friday night, Saturdays, and Sundays, always going to work on Monday morning regardless how sick with a hangover he might have been. On the other hand, Aubrey couldn't stop drinking until the source dried up. Also, they fought. My parents never fought, just argued when he was under the influence until he passed out. Aubrey would break the windows out of her car. My dad never broke a glass or anything.

Their son, Jim, was same age as me. He and I got along pretty good as buddies in school and nobody messed with me or they had to deal with Jim. He did have a little temper, though, and if you messed with him it would come alive. He and I argued over the 620 Kodak Box Camera on a trip to Cherokee I remember and my dad actually bought the camera. He thought it was his.

You would not believe the trip we made to Cherokee, North Carolina, when we were about ten or eleven years old. This was before the Interstate Highway System so you can imagine what the roads were like. Our parents, mine and Jim's, planned the trip and scheduled to leave about nine at night so we would arrive in Cherokee after daylight the next day. Well, that was the first mistake. Our first cousin, Dub, decided to go along too and he agreed to drive Ruby's 1941 Ford. In the front seat was Dub, Ruby, Aubrey, and A.L., Jim's little brother, in Aubrey's lap. In the back seat was my mom, dad, Jim in the left floor board, me in the right floor board, and Sam in mom's lap. It was a ten hour trip across the Blue Ridge Mountains and on to Cherokee in the Great Smoky Mountains with nine of us in that car. Second mistake, dad slipped a pint of juice in mom's pocketbook and, you guessed it, he and Aubrey stayed lit the whole trip.

My mom kept some notes over the years which we found after her passing and in one entry she told of dad and Aubrey taking off one Sunday together and came home late with "two old crooks." That was the only time we know of that he may have crossed the line and one of the few times he was associating with Aubrey.

Chapter 3
Our Other Neighbors

The Owensby family lived several houses down Owl Hill Road below us. They had two sons, one in his early twenty's, and he also drove up and down the road but more conservatively than the rowdy one. I say they had two sons reluctantly because I never saw but one of them ever in the 12 years we were neighbors. The rumor was that son had gotten into some type of trouble as a very young boy and was chained to his bed in the house and was never allowed out of his room, much less outside. The trouble he was being punished for was never publicized, whether it was from stealing, smoking, disrespect, or whatever. It was well known in the neighborhood that he was being held captive by his parents. Everybody talked about it but nobody claims to have seen him.

One day on my way home from school we were walking up the road and about halfway between the Owensby house and ours I looked down where I was walking and there was a $10.00 bill laying right there in the road. I had never held a $10.00 bill before and I knew it was a lot of money. I picked it up and began telling everybody how lucky I was. I was rich in my mind. I had visions of how I was going to spend that much money. It didn't take long, however, for my vision to vanish.

Later that day, after me telling just about everybody I had found

$10.00, there was a knock at our front door. Mom went to the door and it was the Owensby boy stating he understood her son had found "his" $10.00. Of course, we didn't deny the fact that I had found the money. He went on to describe how he had lost it. He said when he got his keys out of his pocket, the money apparently fell out of his pocket and landed on the running board of his car and didn't blow off until he got several yards up the road. Well, that sounded pretty good to my mom so she gave him the money and he went on his way. We never visited this family one time in the 12 years we lived on Owl Hill. They didn't attend our church and you never saw them in town. They just kept to themselves like recluses.

When old man Owensby passed away, it was told that the son being held captive in the house was set free. Of course, no one would be able to recognize him only to say that his skin was white as a sheet and he was skinny as a rail.

It is also strange that no one in the neighborhood questioned this situation or tried to intervene.

Other neighbors included the Barkers. They were old folks as long as I could remember and also stayed out of sight most of the time. He did put out a garden each spring and he used our community mule to do the plowing. Their children were grownups from my beginning and had nothing in common with me or the neighborhood.

Then there were the Holcomb's that lived next to Ruby and Aubrey. They had two sons about mine and Sam's age and we played with them in the sawdust pile and with the toy cars and trucks in the dirt under the big old Oak tree in our yard. Their mom had another baby after they were, it seems like, too far apart.

My first fight was with the oldest Holcomb boy and that was

when I learned something you didn't like had an effect on your ability to think straight and made your blood pressure rise. I said this was a fight but no punches were thrown before it was broken up by my mom. That skirmish had an effect on our relationship thereafter and our friendship was always strained.

The Holcomb's had a pasture almost directly across the road from our house and kept one or two cows for milk. They needed more milk than we did and apparently they liked it better that we did. It was about an acre, rich with green grass and contained with an electric fence all the way around it.

On occasion we would play ball in that pasture and, of course, park our bicycles nearby. One day after our ball playing was over, I jumped on my bicycle and rode through the pasture toward my house. I had completely forgotten about the electric fence and as I approached it, too late, I tried to lower my body to go under but it didn't work. That electric fence caught me across the forehead just above my eyes. I guess I was lucky it didn't hit me in the throat or I would have been hung. I'm not sure whether it was the electric shock or the contact with the fence but it still hurt big time.

Mr. Alex Chatham lived beyond the woods in our back yard in a spectacular house that joined the Hugh Chatham Hospital grounds. He was one of "the" Chatham's and farmed the bottom land along the Yadkin River. He had all these people working for him, mostly black, and we all considered him rich. One of the people working for Mr. Chatham was a black man named Clarence Edwards.

Clarence would drive a team of horses pulling a wagon up and down our road to and from the bottom land farm. He would load it with un-shucked corn or corn stalks used as silage to feed the livestock or whatever the chore of the day would demand.

This man was a people person if there ever was one. He treated all of us kids like his own children and he would let us ride on the wagon which was empty going down and loaded coming back and we thought that was absolutely the most fun you could have. Sometimes the wait would be too long and we would ride one way and have to walk back but it was worth it. I liked Mr. Clarence Edwards.

The McBride's lived across the road from us and this was another family that was different from most normal families. There was old man Tom McBride, his son, Tootsie, his daughter, Ina, and Ina's three kids. I never knew Ina having been married and never knew the father of her three kids.

Herman Laffoon and Bessie lived next to them on Owl Hill. They had three girls, the youngest the same age as me. I liked her a lot too but she never showed me any in return. The two older sisters married brothers and the two brothers were on their way to the Dixie Classic Fair in Winston-Salem one afternoon when their vehicle collided with a working garbage truck and killed both the brothers. A sad time for the Laffoon sisters, both losing their husbands at the same time.

Chapter 4
WE GET EXCITED

Not a lot of excitement happened on Owl Hill except when rowdy wrecked his car or when one of the men would get a little too tipsy on the juice and make a fool of himself. We never saw any law enforcement on Owl Hill. If anything required the law it was handled in town and not at home. Even when Aubrey broke the windows out of Ruby's car she handled it in town and you didn't see any police vehicle or red lights spinning around on top of it.

But that changed one night just after dark. A marked police vehicle pulled into our front yard with its red light flashing and behind it a pickup truck with what looked like a dog's cage and its red light also flashing. We couldn't imagine what was going on and of all things in our front yard.

My dad went outside to investigate and, of course, we were right behind him just as curious. The men in the truck unloaded two big reddish brown dogs with long floppy ears and hung on to them with a long leash. They told my dad they were bloodhounds and a convict had escaped the Wilkes County chain gang and it was believed he might be hiding in the wooded area behind our house. About that time the two men in the truck took off with the two bloodhounds down our driveway into the back yard.

They disappeared into the dark headed toward the woods. When he said convict, I knew what that was. They often worked Owl Hill Road cleaning out the ditches and spreading gravel and all of them wore black and white stripes and their legs were separated by a chain. A man with a long rifle stood nearby guarding them. Hearing this, I headed back into the house and they asked my dad to also go back in and stay inside.

This was in the summertime and the windows were open and we could hear the dogs barking like I had heard Roy's beagles chasing rabbits. They may have been on the trail and they may not have. We never knew if the convict was caught but it was exciting to see that unravel in our front yard.

We were used to hearing sounds of the night since we slept with the windows open so the night breeze would blow through the screen to cool the house after a long hot summer day. Sometimes we would just hook the screen door and actually leave the front and back door open as well to get a better breeze. We never locked our doors even though we had keys. They were the long type about three inches long and I think the keys were called skeleton keys.

We remember the air raids during the war in 1941 and 1942. We called them blackouts. We were supposed to turn out all our lights when the siren sounded from atop Chatham's highest building. We only had one plain old light bulb with a pull string in each room so that was not a hard thing to do. We didn't have lamps because there were no outlets to plug one into.

Looking out the window when the siren would sound towards Chatham's you could watch the lights go out section by section, building by building until it was also dark. This was a scary time for adults and kids like us hung on to mom and dad like glue. We were scared because we had been told an air raid is a warning that we may be under attack from the enemy of the war.

Things like sugar, coffee, metal, and many, many common items you use everyday were rationed and that meant you were limited on how much if any you could purchase from the suppliers. Some of the items required a "ration stamp" which you were issued and if you used all your stamps then you didn't get anymore of that item. Sometimes you had to barter with your friends and neighbors to give them stamps you didn't need for stamps they didn't need in order to manage your situation.

The war not only affected those that were drafted to serve and fight for our country but it also affected those of us left at home in a different way.

Chapter 5
WAS THAT A PANTHER

With the windows open during the summer nights you could hear other sounds as well. After we went to bed and everything was quiet, we could hear the owls, some hoot, hoot and some making sounds like a child crying. There were some of our neighbors who said the owl sounds were not owls but they were from a black panther. They didn't say a bobcat or a cougar, it was a black panther.

I never knew anyone that saw a black panther on Owl Hill but in my mind they did exist in the woods right behind our house.

There were a lot of rabbits and squirrels around as well as possums, skunks, and this was food on the table for us on occasion. My dad built traps for rabbits by nailing four boards together to make a box about three feet long and about six inches wide, enough for a rabbit to enter.

To make it a trap, you had to have a trigger and a door that closed. Dad would take the poker that was used to adjust the coals in the fireplace, and put one end of it in the hottest part of the fire until it was red hot. He would then place the red hot end to the top board of the box and twisting it he could cut a hole in the board for the trigger. He would then do the same for a second hole used to support the door versus. the trigger. We didn't have a drill to bore a hole so this was the next best thing.

After he got the holes like he wanted them, he would make a door and support it with a string to the trigger and anything entering the trap would "throw" it and the door would slam shut.

Once we caught a rabbit dad would pull it out of the box, or rabbit gum as we called it, give it a good lick in the neck to give it a quick death by breaking its neck. He would have me hold the rabbit then by its hind legs and he would begin trimming it with his pocket knife from the part I was holding until he cleared the hind legs. From there you could pull the skin and it would all come off in one piece leaving a clean skinned rabbit. After that he would slit the belly open and remove its insides.

Then mom would take over by cutting off its four legs and splitting the back to make pieces. It would then be boiled until it was tender, fall off the bone tender.

If a possum happened to get trapped in the rabbit gum, dad would burn paper inside the gum to kill the odor. No rabbit will follow a possum into a trap.

We didn't throw away the possum. Dad didn't care for it but mom liked possum. Since they eat practically anything dead, dad would not prepare it immediately to eat. He would put it in a cage and feed it bread and water for several days until in his mind it had cleaned itself inside out.

You have to scald possums to get rid of the hair, remove its head and feet and intestines and then bake it until it is brown and tender. There will be a lot of grease cooked out of the possum when you use this method. The grease is discarded.

We didn't eat squirrels very often. They are too much like a rat but dad did like to take his Remington 22 single shot rifle into the woods and knock one out of a tree once in a while. When you shoot an animal you have to worry about the bullet or "shot' if you are using a shotgun. I don't like biting down on a bullet or shot when eating meat.

Speaking of rats, dad also enjoyed going down to the hog pen and watching for rats and killing them with his old 22 rifle. Where you have hogs, chickens, or any other outside animals you will probably have rats free loading on the food you feed the animals. This was entertainment to him. Some of those rats were really big because they had been eating well.

Our neighbor Roy Chipman always kept two or three beagle dogs and caged them off the ground. I understand this is to sharpen the dog's sense of smell and easier to train for hunting. He didn't do much rabbit hunting but he liked to hear the dogs run and tree raccoons or possums. That type of hunting is done at night and you take your most powerful flashlight with you.

The dogs are kept on a leash until the dogs pick up a scent and then they will want to run and bark to no end. That's when you turn them loose.

You can't keep up with the dogs, you just have to follow their barking and hopefully they tree something soon. I have been with him and my dad possum hunting in the woods behind us. It was thrilling I guess especially for Roy knowing his dogs were trained right but it was thrilling to me too. I looked forward to seeing what the dogs where running which would be my surprise.

If the dogs "treed" the possum or raccoon, they would stop at the base of the tree the animal climbed and continue barking until you shook it down or shot it down. That's when the flashlight comes in to play. You want to see what is in the tree so you shine it in that direction and there you see it, a possum. Mission accomplished.

I have been with them when the dogs picked up a scent and then would be turned loose to run. In a few cases, if the dogs didn't tree anything they would keep running and barking and it might be the next day before the dogs show up back at home. They always did come home, though, tired and hungry and then be put back in the elevated cages until the next time. Often during these nights we would see an owl or two.

The Yadkin River ran through Elkin from west to east and parallel to the railroad tracks and Highway 268 where the entrance to Owl Hill was. Occasionally when we would have heavy rains the river would flood and do tremendous damage in Elkin. In 1940, before they built the Yadkin River Dam in North Wilkesboro, North Carolina, we had the granddaddy flood of all time. I remember mom leading me down Owl Hill Road toward Highway 268 with a whole lot of other people to see the flood. The river had covered the Chatham Blanketeer's Ball Park, covered the railroad tracks, and covered Highway 268. As we approached the waters edge, we climbed a bank up to Finn Haynes' house, walked across his yard to the East Elkin Baptist Church and stood on the front steps of the church watching the enormous amount of water. The water covered the church parking lot. A huge oil tank had broken loose from the force of the water somewhere up stream and when it hit the electric wires it exploded in a big fire. This fire was on top of the water and flowing down stream making a spectacular site to see.

Chapter 6
GRANDPA GENTRY'S HOUSE

Decatur Gentry was my grandpa on my mom's side and a visit to his house was a real treat for a little kid like me. He and his first wife, Fostina (Tina) Darnell, had five children, Opal, my mom, Famie, Ruby, Fairy, and Omar. When mom was nine years old, Tina died from pneumonia. He remarried this time to Annie Mounce. They had four children, Marie, Clifford, Toledo, and Geneva. That was a total of nine children. And, he still lived to marry three more times. It would be up to mom to get someone to drive us down there and once there grandpa would usually bring us back home. At his house we could play in the barn loft where he kept the hay for his horses, Dixie and Dan. We could see chickens and look for eggs in the hen's nest and take them to Grandma Annie. We could see her milk the cow and kill a chicken for dinner. We could play on the tractors and sometimes they would take us for a ride on the tractors. Sometimes grandpa would hook the horses up to the wagon and take us for a ride. It was always fun at grandpa's house.

If we went to visit on Saturday he would often be at the saw mill. Grandma would tell where he was working and I would walk down there just to watch that big round saw blade saw through a tree two or three feet thick. The first run of the saw was the throwaways or slabs as they are called. My dad built his pig pens out of slabs.

Grandpa had a lot of people working for him and he provided them with a shack to live in. Most of them were paid in cash minus the juice he provided them for the weekends. One man in particular had a real bad limp, one leg was shorter than the other one. His nickname was "step and a half."

The other business my Grandpa Gentry was involved in was white lightning. He had a lot of visitors when we were there but never saw the transaction take place. He took them out to the shed on the other side of the hedges from the house. Grandpa Gentry also had two big white horses he used on the farm. One of the horse's name was Dixie and the other one was Dan. Mom told us of the time Dan was sick and she and grandpa sat up with the horse all night. She remembered old Dan lying on its side in the barn with his head propped on the door sill until he finally passed away. It was a tragic time for her and grandpa because she said he really loved those two horses and had owned them for a long time.

My dad didn't go with us to visit Grandpa Gentry very often. He didn't share his juice and never saw him drink it. It was a business for him. That meant my dad would have to "visit" like mom was doing.

Problem was, though, when we did get back home after our visit dad would be high as a kite and we would have to put up with that again. It seems like Grandpa Gentry would have learned his lesson in dealing with moonshine. Some years before I was born he was charged with bootlegging and sent to the Atlanta Prison. Mom had letters from him while he was there telling them he was doing okay and for them to help mama for him while he was gone.

He did learn a trade while in prison, though, and that was carpentry and working with wood. That trade was converted to saw milling after he came home and was quite a respectable business for him.

It was my understanding he was there while they were building the railroad into the prison for the transfer of Al Capone.

Grandpa's tractor that he used for the fields was an awesome one with great big iron rear wheels that had cleats instead of tires and the front wheels were also iron with no tires. The tractor that he used at the saw mill to pull the blade was a more modern one with tires. It had a pulley to one side of the engine and a long belt ran from there to the pulley on the shaft of the saw blade. When you started the tractor, you could put it in gear and the pulley would start turning the saw.

Once during our visit to grandpa's house some men were hand digging a well at the tenant house. The hole at the time looked to be about twenty to twenty-five feet deep. One of the men had a rope looped around his waist and legs and was lowered by the other men into the hole. Then another rope was used to lower a bucket, short handle pick, and a short handle shovel. When the man in the hole filled the bucket with dirt, the others would pull the bucket up and empty it and lower it back down for him to fill it up again. The oxygen level and the backbreaking work for one man would not last long so they would rotate to give each other a break.

When the digging struck a water vein and it was big enough to fill the bottom of the hole, that part was finished. They would then build a wooden box over the hole and center a bucket tied to a rope over the hole so when they lowered this bucket it would fill with water and being lowered over the hole would not rub the dirt walls of the hole to muddy the fresh water being pulled up. It was always good to visit Grandpa Gentry's house and see my grandma use an ax and chop the head off a chicken and then clean that chicken and make a big pot of chicken stew with dumplings to feed us all that day.

My great grandpa was Allech Woddston Gentry and he was married to Jurandy Marshall. He died in 1937, the year I was born. Going back a little further in my research some names appeared directly from the bible and I thought it a little odd. For example, back in 1761 there was a Meshack Gentry married to Ann. They lived in Virginia and North Carolina, died in Monroe, Tennessee. The strangest part is he had two brothers, one named Shadrach and the other one Obednego Gentry. Old Allech and Jurandy must have been reading the bible.

My great-great grandpa was Austin Gentry. He was married to Mahalia Crouse. He was born in 1827 and died in 1899, the year of my dads' birth. Austin has a little history attached to his name. He was a soldier in the 37th NC Regiment, Company F. He signed on in Wilkesboro, North Carolina, with the Carolina Western Stars. The militia moved to High Point, North Carolina, and then to Raleigh. There it was integrated into the Confederate Army Company F of the 37th NC Regiment.

This unit fought at New Bern, then became part of the Army of Northern Virginia, General Lee's Army, and was part of a Brigade of North Carolina troops in AP Hill's Division in Stonewall Jackson's II Corps. They saw action in all the major battles. Austin was captured April 2nd outside Petersburg, Virginia. The Regiment surrendered with Lee at Appomattox on April 9, 1865. He was paroled from Point Lookout, Maryland, in July 1865.

Chapter 7

GRANDPA HINSON'S HOUSE

My Grandpa Hinson was named Charlie Columbus Hinson. He passed away from the gangrene poison and I can barely remember him. The picture in my mind is the one of him sitting in the doorway of his bedroom, which led to the wrap around porch. He and his wife, Nancy Cockerham Hinson, had, in addition to my dad, his twin brother Dewey, Claude, Guy, Warrick, and a sister named Elma. Mom said they all sipped the juice, even the sister Elma. Warrick and his wife, Callie, always lived with grandpa, even after he got married and raised his own family. He still lived in the old home place until he died from natural causes as an old man. We didn't visit them as much as my Grandpa Gentry because it was more difficult to get someone to come get us and bring us back home. You see, my mom usually made all the arrangements, so she favored going where she wanted to go and it worked to her advantage.

One thing I learned quickly visiting Warrick, you don't walk through a fresh cut field of wheat barefooted even to get to ride on the wagon. The wheat stubble will bring the blood to your feet since I was usually barefooted in the summer time. Warrick raised mostly wheat and rye and corn on their farmland and used a team of horses to pull most of the equipment utilized in planting and harvesting the crops. They didn't have a tractor that I remember, not even one with the big iron wheels with cleats instead of tires.

Warrick and his wife, Callie, had several children, Ira, Herman, twins Connie and Lonnie, Ruby and Bobby. Bobby was just a little older than me and sometimes when we were visiting he would take me down to the creek that drew the line of their property and their next farmland neighbor. I had seen clay that you buy in the Dime Store, but this creek had a bank of clay and Bobby would show me how to dislodge it and mold it into an object and when that object dried, it would be gray and hard as a brick. Warrick used this clay to seal the front of their rock fire places. They had one in every bedroom. I am sure they used it for other reasons but this one stood out in my mind.

When Warrick saw us coming into the house on a visit he never failed to say "here come them Republicans."

Dad's twin brother, Dewey, and his wife had twelve children and all twelve were girls. Not one boy. Two of the girls were twins, Ima and Nina, and for some reason Warrick raised them when Dewey and his wife and the other ten children moved to Danville, Virginia.

After several years living in Danville, all his girls had married, but not all of them moved out. He gained a son in some cases so he continued to have a big family. One night, all the children and husbands and grandkids were out of the house. This hardly ever occurred with such a large family and just the two of them were at home, Dewey and his wife.

In the quiet of the night, a gun shot rung out in the bedroom adjacent to where they were just sitting. Dewey had gotten up and went into the bedroom and there he lay, dead from a "self inflicted gunshot wound." No warning, no argument, no drinking, no kids at home, and no reason could be given by the family.

Nina, Dewey's daughter that Warrick raised, and husband Paul asked my dad if he would like to go to Danville to the funeral with him and Nina and if so he could ride in the back of his open bed pickup. It was summertime and he had a tarp in case it rained. So, my dad agreed to go and mom, me, and Sam also went, all riding in the back of a pickup truck all the way from Elkin, North Carolina, to Danville, Virginia. We used two of our cane bottom chairs for mom and dad to sit on and Sam and I sat on a blanket.

Fortunately, it didn't rain and thankfully was not too hot.

That must have been the first funeral I had been to, even though we went to East Elkin Baptist Church on a regular basis. I am sure there were other funerals held there over time but I believe this was my first one.

Since all of Dewey's children were girls, they disappeared by way of marriage using their husbands name and we lost all contact with all of them except the two that Warrick and Callie raised, Ima and Nina. Both of them and their husbands settled in Wilkes County at the foot of the Blue Ridge Mountains very near my Grandpa Hinson's farmland. We always laughed at the Hinson's ending up at the foot of the Blue Ridge Mountains. We decided that their migration from Jamestown, Virginia, was west but getting over the mountain was just too much, so that's where they settled down, Wilkes County, North Carolina, with the mountain in their background.

My great Grandfather Parm Hinson was a more interesting Hinson relative than most. He was born in 1852 in Stanley County, North Carolina, and reportedly died in Cleburne, Texas, and buried in the Cleburne Memorial Cemetery. He was married to Mary

McCann who was born in 1855, in State Road, Traphill Township, Wilkes County, North Carolina. Parm and Mary had seven children, one being Charles Columbus Hinson, my grandpa.

Its been told Mary's sister, Rebecca McCann, came to live with Parm and Mary to finish school and Parm must had fallen in love with Rebecca so the two of them packed the wagon and left town together. Parm had promised one of his sons, John Martin, he would bring him a Case Knife when he returned. They never returned. His wife, Mary, gave birth to a child after Parm left that obviously was not Parm's. She was given the last name Yale.

Parm and Rebecca married or not and went on to have six children of their own. To add a little history to the Hinson family, my great-great grandpa was Martin Hinson who was born in 1823 in Stanly County, North Carolina, and was married to Martha. This marriage produced seven kids. There was Franklin, Julia, Saphrona, Parm (my great grandpa), Ephraim, Giles, and Ann.

Going back to about 1756, my great-great-great grandpa was Samuel Hinson. He was born in Culpepper County, Virginia, and died October 22, 1844, in Stanly County, North Carolina. He turned 20 at the start of the Revolutionary War. It is not clear when he married, but according to the census of 1800 he was left with seven children and no wife shown. He lived in Virginia at the time and may have served in the war. By the time of the War of 1812 he was a lone parent probably still taking care of the children on his farm. His residence on January 1788 was 200 acres in Chatham County, North Carolina. This parcel of land is described as situated lying and being in the County and State beginning at a pine on Jeremiah Melton's line at Browns Corner and running west eighty two poles to a post oak then south twenty two poles to a pine at Urdeman's Corner then down his line south forty five degrees west one hundred and twenty six poles to a pine then west twenty poles to a pine then south ninety three poles to a pine west line then along said line south sixty degrees east six poles to a pine then east one hundred and eighty eight poles to a post oak then north two hundred and ten poles to the first station including estimation two hundred acres of land.

One of the things my family and I really enjoyed was a trip up the Blue Ridge Mountains to the Blue Ridge Parkway and taking a picnic lunch to Wildcat Rock, Cumberland Knob, or the many other perfect places for a picnic. On a clear day you could see the Hinson farm area from the top of the mountain. Usually it was a blanket on the ground type picnic with the women bringing the home cooked food and, of course, always a watermelon. So, anytime we could get someone to go on a picnic we were always ready. We were so dependent on someone else since my dad never drove or owned another car after the T-Model. Mom was glad because of his drinking.

These events were sometimes with the Chipman family, but mostly with one of my uncles and aunts. We would eat till we were about to pop and then walk some of the trails that were scattered through the Blue Ridge Parkway, come back and eat watermelon.

We would also go to Stone Mountain State Park for the view of this big majestic boulder sticking several hundred feet out of the ground, a big round oval shaped rock, and watch the brave souls that practiced rock climbing do their stuff. Sometimes we would pick chinquapins, chestnuts, and gooseberries. In season we would buy a sack of mountain cabbage to make kraut. Mountain apples were a must buy. We would always play in the cool waters of the mountain streams full of stocked trout supplied by the fisheries located at the top of the mountain. The fisheries were always a favorite of mine just to see the process from fish eggs hatching in these containers, a step up was the next stage of the fish growth all the way to the outside ponds holding the trout to be shipped to the various mountain streams in the area. I never went fishing as a kid.

Chapter 8
GROWING UP ON OWL HILL

When I reached the age to go to school, we only had one choice in Elkin City Schools and that was Elkin Elementary School which was located almost in town but at the top of a real steep hill. There were no school buses traveling Owl Hill Road so we had to walk the approximately one and one half miles down the crooked, gravel, dirt road, turn right on Highway 268, which was Main Street, proceed through downtown and up the steep hill to the top. We usually walked in groups from the area, two or three or more together rather than alone. If it was raining, one of the neighbors would drive a group of us and sometimes we used the Chipman's telephone to call a cab and our parents would split the fare.

My lunch was often a homemade biscuit with a piece of pork or maybe just a mayonnaise biscuit. I would carry it in my overalls pocket because we didn't have lunch bags. My dad took his lunch in a lunch bucket that had a thermos but that would be too much expected of me to take to school. Mom was instructed by my dad to cook breakfast and supper every day and always lunch on Sunday. He wanted fresh biscuits morning and night with his meals. He bought flour in twenty-five pound bags. Breakfast was usually sausage and eggs or country ham and eggs and cream gravy and biscuits. Sometimes Sam and I would eat corn flakes for breakfast but I had a problem of spilling mine. Corn flakes were served to us in a drinking glass, not a bowl, and for me they were real easy to spill. We always had syrup and real butter on the table for the biscuits as well. Supper was usually boiled pork meat and potatoes, green beans, or black eye peas, corn, turnips, turnip greens, pintos, tomatoes, and etc., and biscuits. Sunday lunch was usually stewed chicken, chicken gravy, and dumplings. We never had loaf bread, corn bread, beef of any kind, tea, soft drinks, hot dogs or hamburgers.

I always wore overalls to school even though a lot of my clothes were made by my mom. She learned to sew early in life and made a lot of our clothes. Once when my dad had bought me a brand new pair of overalls at Smithy's Store I decided to leave the label on the bib so everybody would know I had on new overalls and was no slouch with home made clothes. Well, that kind of backfired. The first one that noticed wanted to know if they were not paid for and I couldn't take the tag off until they were. The tag came off promptly. My shoes were Keds high top tennis shoes.

On a very cold morning sometimes we would stop by W. W. Whitakers Grocery Stores right in the center of town and warm by the big pot belly stove located in the center of the store. A lot of old men would be doing the same thing before proceeding on their way to work or wherever. One of these old men, on one of the coldest mornings ever, grabbed my nearly frozen ear and twisted it wanting to know is your ears cold. I thought my ear was about torn from my head and it hurt all day.

Since we had no hot water except heating it on the kitchen stove or using the water tank attached to the stove, we often went without bathing for long periods of time. In hindsight, I can remember my feet were rusty from going barefooted and then put on clean socks and shoes over the dirty feet. I can remember getting rusty on my neck behind my ears and I never brushed my teeth. We were not taught any different and thought it was absolutely normal. When I got a little older I had a tooth to break off and mom took me to see Dr. Fox., the local dentist. I can remember he said I wouldn't have a tooth in my head by the time I was grown from rot. I was lucky though, I took him seriously and actually only lost four by taking better care of them. I also started heating my own water and washing up more often after I started noticing everybody was not rusty. It hurts when one of your peers calls you rusty to your face.

I didn't like school and sometimes I would go to the schoolhouse and then leave without going inside. I would spend the day in the railroad yard sometimes just sitting in one of the open boxcars sitting idle on the tracks. It was my idea of being a hobo and I thought seriously about that being my next move in life. I would be a hobo and travel everywhere the train goes.

Sometimes I would steal one of the bicycles from the bicycle rack at school and just ride it around all day and take it back before school let out but I got caught doing that. That day my third grade teacher, Mrs. Rhinehart, was waiting on me and boy did I get a lecture. That wasn't all I got when I got home. My dad had a leather strap that he used to sharpen his razor blade and it had three holes in one end of it. That leather strap left three blisters everywhere it struck my behind and there were a lot.

My dad was drinking a lot now and my mom was taking a lot of verbal abuse from him and I hated the arguing, mouthing, and slobbering until he passed out. Many times when he couldn't get off the couch, let alone stand up, he would beg me to shoot him if he would get his rifle down for me. He didn't beg mom to shoot him, he didn't beg Sam to shoot him, it was always me. I was old enough to know better and considering the condition he was is in. It really hurt to hear him say shoot me. Sometimes mom would take Sam and me outside and just walk around the yard until we could no longer hear him mouthing. So, I decided one day I would leave home and I did. I rode my bicycle the five miles to my Grandpa Gentry's house and spent the day at his house but he thought it best I go back home so he arranged that. That old leather strap found my behind again, leaving three blisters everywhere those three holes hit.

Then it happened, the big surprise and shock to Owl Hill. Chatham's had notified all its tenants on Owl Hill that they would have to move. Chatham's wanted to expand into the area and the tenants would have to go. They said, you can have the house, you can move it to your own private lot, you can tear it down and salvage any parts you wish, or you can simply abandon as is. You just have to get out of the area. That started a lot of people scrambling because $4.32 monthly rent doesn't give you much incentive to relocate. I remember Henry Bowman bought a piece of land and moved his house. He was the only one. Everyone else either abandoned or salvaged what they could. That was the worst thing for my dad because he had no sense of direction to take, no money to work with, and no idea what his next step would be. Mom had always taken the lead when the chips were down so what could mom do now. This was in 1948-1949 and I was twelve going on thirteen, Sam was three years younger and Charlie was on his own in and out.

Funny thing, Chatham's had just built a bathroom in all of the tenant houses. There was no hot water but we didn't have to take the path down to the outhouse anymore or clean the slop jar the next morning.

Chapter 9

Johnson Ridge

One of mom's sisters was named Famie. Her husband was Willie Phillips. Willie was another Aubrey. They had six kids, Garvey, Bill, Dub, Bob, Doris, and Lydia. I never knew Willie to work public work and I could never tell if he was sober or drunk because he acted the same all the time, drunk. She lived on Johnson Ridge Road and it was about two miles east of where we were on Owl Hill. It was a dirt gravel road with pasture belonging to Elkin's richest man, Andrew Greenwood, on both sides leading up the hill from Highway 268. I actually killed one of Mr. Greenwood's registered white face heifers with my car one day going up Johnson Ridge. They used the road like a cow lane to drive cattle since Mr. Greenwood owned the land and had pastures on both sides of the road for a half mile or so. They claimed they were driving the heifer from one pasture to the other and it darted out from behind their jeep and actually hit my car broadside in the left front fender and driver's side door. The people working for Mr. Greenwood claimed I was speeding and my insurance company ended up paying him for the accident. Their word against a 16-17 year old boy ruled.

Famie had worked for Chatham's in the past and had built her little house some years earlier. She had also moved to Winston-Salem for a period and worked at the famous Robert E. Lee Hotel as a house keeper but had moved back to this house after Willie passed away. Three of her children still lived with her and her oldest son, Garvey, had built a house next to her. The land beyond Garvey was vacant and caught mom's eyes for two reasons. One, we had to move and two, it was next to her sister if she could find the owner and be able to purchase enough land to build us a house. It took a while but she finally located the owner, Frank Ryecroft, and he agreed to sell her one acre for $300.00 adjacent to Garvey's house. She went straight to Franklin Folger, President of The Bank of Elkin, and borrowed the $300.00 and immediately became a land owner.

Mr. Folger was always friendly and professional and he would let my mom have a hundred, two hundred, whatever when she wanted to buy a new couch, mattress, and etc., and pay it back $10.00 a week or even $5.00 a week. She was a good credit risk and made small loans occasionally over the years. The next step was to agree on a house plan and get it under construction just as soon as possible. She was ready to leave Owl Hill and hoped that it would have an improved effect on dad's drinking.

Mom had always been active in the church and at a point in time so was my dad. Mom, however, got involved in the First Baptist Church of Elkin during the short time they lived on Cotton Mill Hill which was just behind the Elkin Elementary School and walking distance to the church. This is actually where my older brother, Charlie, was born. This was the church the upper society people of Elkin attended and my dad didn't feel comfortable going there so she went alone. When they moved to Owl Hill, they went to East Elkin Baptist Church and he would attend with her on occasion. The problem was, mom had ties to the First Baptist Church and tried to attend both as much as possible.

At the First Baptist Church mom was a Program Leader of the WMU, (Women's Missionary Unit), two years, Community Mission, she was Chairman two years, and President of the WMU for five years. It was difficult to leave that responsibility but the membership was declining and it was a long ways to walk to and from and East Elkin Baptist Church was closer so East Elkin Baptist Church won out for her membership. That was more my dad's kind of church and he would attend with her when he was not sipping the juice that weekend. I was also saved one night during the Wednesday night prayer meets and was baptized at East Elkin Baptist Church in Elkin, North Carolina. I was about 12 years old. Prayer meeting was held in different member's homes on Wednesday nights and not in the church as they are today.

Building a house and moving to Johnson Ridge would be a couple miles from East Elkin Church so that was going to be a problem but mom was glad to be getting away from Owl Hill and all the drinking and would cross that bridge when she got to it.

Mom kept urging dad to get moving on the construction but he was not a leader and he didn't know where to start. So, mom asked Roy if he would help us out since he was a supervisor of carpentry at Chatham's and he had a lot of experience and contacts. Over a few drinks with dad he agreed to give it a shot and helped us out even though he was one of the reasons mom wanted to leave Owl Hill so badly. He was such a bad influence on dad she thought with his drinking. Roy could handle his better than dad could and it showed.

Roy got the ball rolling and told dad to get him $1500.00 and he would get the work started. He hired Lester Haynes to dig, pour, and lay the foundation blocks. He made arrangements to get salvage lumber from some of the abandoned houses for the sub-flooring and roof sheathing. He and his friends built the framing and rafters from Thurman Lumber Yard. Charlie was working evening shift and he would be there sometimes at 7:30AM to help. Clarence Foote then came in and built the chimneys and fireplace. Most of the interior doors came from one or more of the abandoned houses. All of these people worked as friends and social drinking associates thanks to Roy Chipman. I was only 12 but mom and I with a little help from Sam picked up the scrap lumber and piled it neatly for future use in the kitchen stove and fireplace. Nothing at all was thrown away.

On July 2, 1949, we moved into our new house leaving Owl Hill for the owls, black panthers, and Chatham's expansion.. The hearth for the fireplace was not finished and we laid boards across the hole to avoid stepping in it and falling into the crawl space. That's when we saw a snake crawling between the boards going into the crawl space from our living room. Shortly after that one was found behind the couch in the living room, apparently coming through between the boards over where the hearth would eventually be. That one was killed and it turned out to be a black snake. From then on we would often find black snake skins hanging on the cinder blocks in the crawl space. Apparently we built a house over a black snake's territory and they didn't leave.

We had a well drilled for our water and it became very expensive, 300 feet deep. A pump was put in the crawl space so we had running water but, again, no hot water. As time passed, though, we did get a hot water heater, an electric stove, refrigerator, and an oil circulator to heat the three bedrooms, bathroom, kitchen, dining room and living room. Thanks to Roy and all the talented people he knew for each project they chipped in to make this happen with so little money and so little leadership from my dad. Thanks to the man my mom had grown tired of his bragging and his influence on dad. Charlie got married to Nell Johnson from Taylorsville, North Carolina, about this time so the little transportation he had provided now dwindled to nothing.

We still depended on our friends and neighbors and City Cabs to take us anywhere we needed to go. Dad made arrangements with Stella Bauguss to ride to work with her since she also worked at Chatham's. Later on in years he rode with her son, Howard Bauguss, and then it was Cal Griffin. On occasion there was no one conveniently available and he would walk the two miles to work. We were fortunate, though, a school bus traveled Johnson Ridge and we got to ride the bus to Middle School for the next two years. After that we rode the bus to Elkin High School as well. Bernard Jackson was the bus driver. Clarence Swaim, the kid that shoved my wagon off the Walkers porch to its demise when I was three years old, was now our new neighbor again. He lived in the next house past the several acres of vacant land between us. The move didn't improve my dad's drinking habit at all. It only introduced him to a new group of juice sipping friends. He was always able to work but weekends would be hard to take. Why he mouthed so much at my mom I don't know, but I often wonder if she must have given him a reason at some point early in the marriage and he never forgave or forgot.

Chapter 10

FAMIE'S SAGA

Famie's oldest son, Garvey, that lived next door was in the bootlegging business with his younger brother, Bobby. That was an easy source for dad's moonshine because it was next door and provided additional sales for Garvey for dad's social drinking friends as well. Junior Johnson didn't have a thing on Garvey and Bob, they were doing the same thing, building hot rod 40 Fords, 34 Fords with Elderbloch headers, and Columbia rear ends that would exceed 100 miles an hour easily. They would take the floor boards out of the vehicles and put braces in to lower and increase the size of the interior to hold more cases of moonshine. The divider between the car's trunk and the back seat or front seat with the coupes would also be removed to make more room. Sometimes they would be chased by the law enforcement and get away and on occasion there would be a wreck but no one ever was hurt and got away. I helped Bill one year when he was raising tobacco. My job was to drive the tractor and pull the sleds from the field to the barn where it was being processed to go into the barn for curing. I was about fourteen or fifteen, no driver's license, but they asked me to go to the store and get some cold drinks for all of them. He told me to drive the 34 Ford sedan that was parked at the barn and be careful. Well, I could drive a tractor but didn't have any experience in driving a car and this car was special. When I put it in first gear and let the clutch out, the seat went backwards. It wasn't bolted down and I could see the ground below me because the floor boards had been removed. Finally, I recovered and started again and when I did this time, a pistol fell into my lap from the sun visor above. This was one of the bootlegging cars and I was driving it to the store to get everybody a cold Pepsi.

When Interstate 77 was being constructed across the Yadkin River into Surry County, it temporarily ended at the intersection of Highway 21 north, just inside the county. The grading had extended for several miles but no paving yet. About fifteen hundred feet from the end of the pavement there was a drop off down an embankment into a wooded area. It also had a stream running parallel with I-77. Being in the area frequently going up Highway 21 it was noticeable there were vehicle tracks extending into the dirt area. These tracks were a dead giveaway that somebody was visiting that area. Actually, somebody had built themselves a moonshine liquor still on that little stream in the woods and just off the uncompleted I-77. When it was busted up by the ATF people, it was almost like a tourist attraction for everybody including me. I was able to see a real liquor still even though it was busted up. Nobody was ever arrested but it was awfully close to where Garvey and Bob lived on Johnson Ridge.

These two idiots Garvey and Bob had never worked a day in their life at public work and then got greedy and started stealing things to pawn or sell to keep their business thriving. The greed got them caught and they were both sent to prison for a spell. When they were released, Garvey and his wife, Helen, moved to Lenoir, North Carolina, supposedly looking for public work. Bob took a job driving a tractor and trailer across country, from North Carolina to

California. I heard he was also hauling drugs out of Mexico with his cargo in fake panels in the trailer.

Everybody knew corn liquor, or white lightning, was illegal and everybody that indulged in it had their own way of hiding it. Famie had wooden boards laid down on her path to the outhouse to keep from stepping in the mud. Her husband, Willie, would take the posthole digger and dig a hole underneath one of these boards and store maybe three or four jars of white liquor in the hole, then replace the board and never know it was there.

The house Garvey built next door to his mom had grooved knotty pine panels in the living room. He built these panels so that they would slide up into the ceiling, store his juice and then lower the panel. Who would know that the panels would slide up and down and hide such an item. My dad just hid his in a paper bag in his bedroom closet.

Garvey and Helen's move to the Lenoir area was apparently the breaking up of him and Bob's illegal activities and we heard Garvey had settled down out in the country and was raising hogs. It was hog killing time and Garvey was taking advantage of the season and preparing one of his hogs for slaughter out back of his house just like my dad used to do. For some strange and unorthodox reason, Garvey pulled the liver from the hog's stomach cavity and took it into the house. Inside, he took the wet, bloody liver and dropped it in Helen's lap while she was sitting in a living room chair for no apparent reason that we knew of or heard about. It was just like someone simply lost it.

Helen was furious and went into the next room, pulled out a family pistol and sat back down in the chair with the gun in her lap and a newspaper hiding it from sight. When Garvey walked back into the room, BAM, Helen fired the pistol killing Garvey instantly.

This, of course, was very hard on Famie, his mom, my mom's sister, and she was very distraught over the tragedy as you would imagine.

Bob was still driving a tractor/trailer and was saving up to buy a truck of his own and lease out instead of driving a company provided one. This would enable him to make more money and be more independent. I heard he had saved up $30,000 cash and Famie was holding the money for him. Some said he was about ready to make the deal. And then there was another shocker. Bob was found dead, rolled up in a rug, on the front porch of his girlfriend's house with a fatal bullet to the back of his head. Both boys were now dead from gunshot wounds, both murdered, both lived by the sword and both died by the sword. His killer was never identified.

A short time later mom went to Famie's early one morning as she did often since she moved two doors away and the front door was unlocked, which was not uncommon. Mom went inside calling Famie by name but there was no answer. She went into the bedroom and Famie was still in bed. Mom took Famie's hand to arouse her and found it dead cold. The ambulance was called and when they uncovered her, she had a bullet hole in her chest, hardly any blood, and a small pistol laying by her side. She was pronounced dead from a self-inflicted gunshot wound. Or was it self inflicted? Did Bob's $30,000 have anything to do with her death? We will never know but it does raise questions in my mind.

Mom's youngest sister was Fairy. She was married to William Cooper. They were in the restaurant business for many years. William actually was the cook at some popular restaurants in Winston-Salem at one time. One of those was Manuel's Restaurant on 4th Street downtown. He later owned and operated his own restaurant on Hawthorne Road adjacent to the Wake Forest Baptist Hospital. He lived in Winston-Salem at times and at other times he commuted to Winston-Salem from Elkin where he stayed in the home he owned next door to my Grandpa Gentry. The point of mentioning William and Fairy is the inspiration he had on me and most others that knew him in his golden years. William was a diabetic and after he retired from the restaurant business and moved back to Elkin for good he lost a leg from his condition which was removed at the knee. Sometime later the other leg became infected and it had to be removed at the hip. He had an artificial leg he could use on the leg removed at the knee so with one leg on the ground per sey, he could still get around with crutches somewhat but barely.

The inspiration part comes when garden planting season comes around. William had a Farmall tractor and when he strapped the artificial leg on he could actually mount that tractor and plow his garden using the artificial leg to operate the foot pedals. But it doesn't end there. He modified a riding lawnmower that he could ride through the garden and use a hoe to lay off the rows, plant the garden, and weed it all the time on the modified riding lawnmower. At harvest time he would mount the riding lawnmower and ride the rows and harvest his crops. How many people do you know that has lost both legs and still plants a garden?

William and Fairy sometimes carried us back home after visiting Grandpa Gentry since they lived next door and I can also remember them taking us on trips to the mountains in his Model A Ford when I was just a little tyke.

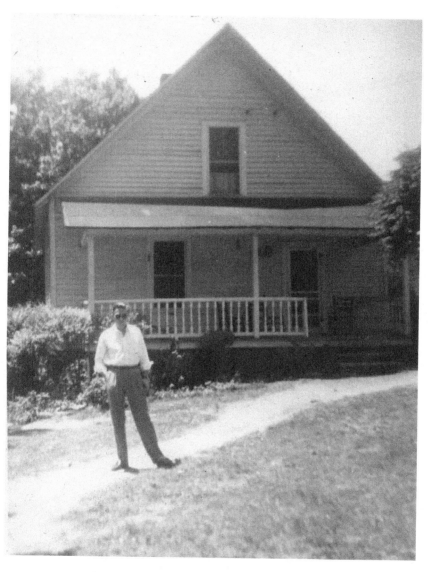

Owl Hill Home place and older brother Charlie Hinson

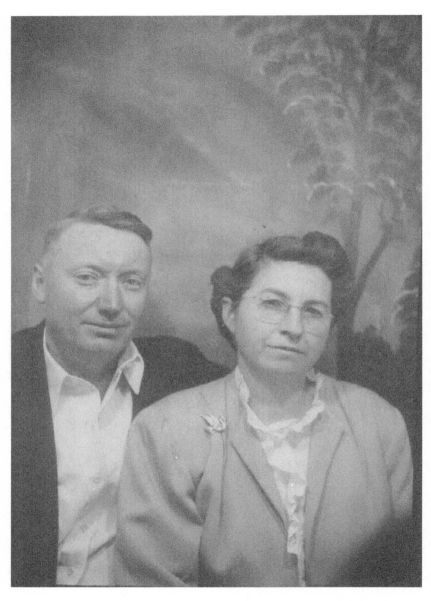

Mom and Dad - Winfield Shelly Hinson and Opal Ophelia Gentry Hinson

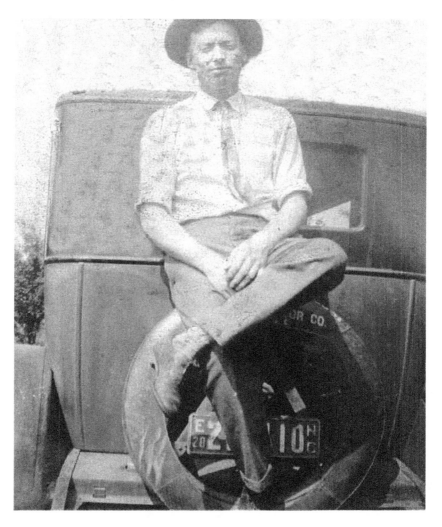

Dad and the only car he ever owned

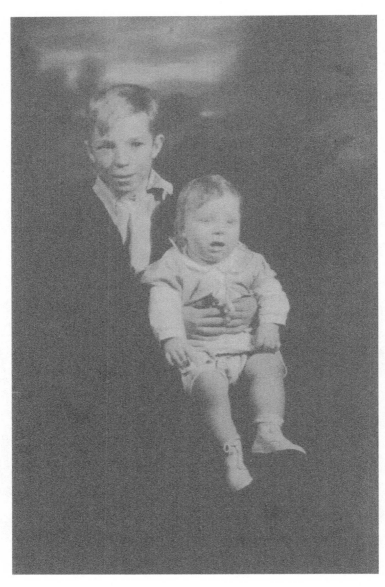

Charlie Hinson with Harold Hinson on his lap

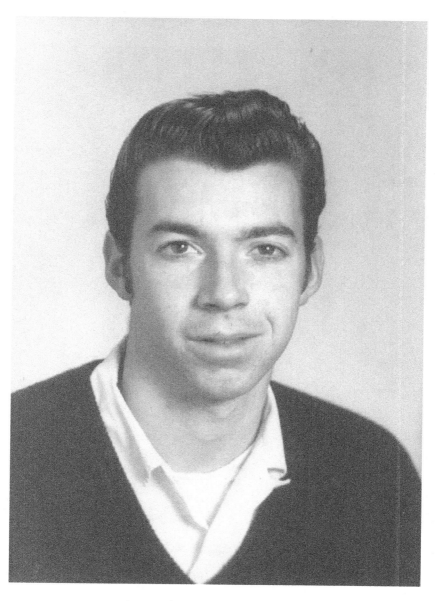

Younger brother Samuel Lee Hinson

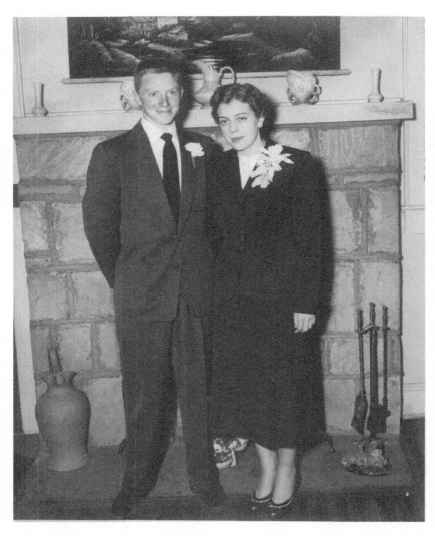

Harold Hinson and Faye Wilmoth Hinson Wedding April 16, 1954

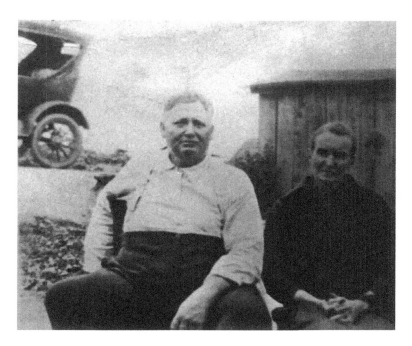

Grandparents Charlie Columbus Hinson and Nancy Cockerham Hinson

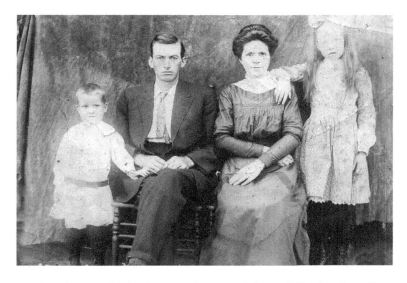

*Grandparents Risdon Decatur Gentry and first wife Fostina Darnell
Gentry with son Omar on left and daughter Famie on right*

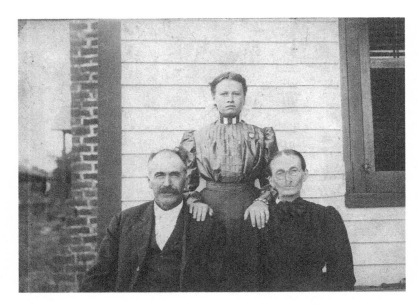

Great Grand Parents Allech Gentry and Jurandy Gentry with daughter Sally

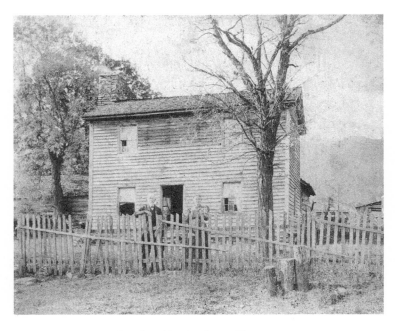

Grandma Fostina Darnell's parents

Chapter 11
My First Job

The move to Johnson Ridge turns out was a big change in my life. I was 13-14 years old and Charlie was managing the Valley Drive Inn Theater in Jonesville and other jobs right before he married Nell but when he slept, he was usually at home. He had gone to work one afternoon and was getting ready for the evening show. The boy that sold popcorn and drinks to the cars parked in the field didn't show up and Charlie came back home to get me to help them out. I was glad to do so. This was a night job and didn't interfere with school and I was going to get paid.

Charlie showed me what I was supposed to do and I began packing the drink wagon with Pepsi Colas on ice and popcorn in a separate area. I waited for the time to start my round to visit each car parked in the drive-inn to offer my hot popcorn and cold drinks. Boy, I must have put too many drinks in the wagon because it was really heavy and hard to push. The drive-inn lot was a gravel lot, not paved, so I had my work cut out for me. I did survive the first night, though, and it became my regular job. I learned not to pack so many drinks on the next round and repacked for the second run through the field. I would ride back and forth home with Charlie or Dub, one of Famie's boys who lived with his mom and also worked there, or a friend that happened to be around.

Finally, I was "promoted" to popping popcorn in the office, keeping the drink cooler filled, cleaning up after closing, etc., and someone else was hired to push that drink cart. But, shortly after that the projectionist, Bud Durham, who was a "bleeder" was involved in an auto accident trying to dodge a dog in the road and later passed away. After I finished my duties popping popcorn and etc., I would hang around in the projection booth with Bud. His work sparked my attention and he would sometimes let me switch reels so I could get the feel of it. By the time of his accident, I could do most of the projectionist duties or was aware of how to do it even if I had never performed it. As a result of this gain of knowledge, I became the projectionist.

My junior year in high school I was allowed to take diversified education class and was given credit for working. On my sixteenth birthday I got my driver's license and started immediately looking for a car. I had saved two hundred dollars and it was deposited in The Bank of Elkin. Since mom had such a good relationship with Franklin Folger, I mustered up the nerve to visit him and ask for a loan. Mr. Folger asked me what I wanted to do with a loan and I told him I wanted to buy a car. He then asked how old are you and I replied sixteen. He said then you aren't old enough to own a car so he had to deny my request for a loan. I told him that it was okay, just give me my two hundred dollars and I would go find me a two hundred dollar car and that is exactly what I did. I never patronized The Bank of Elkin ever again.

I found a two hundred dollar 1941 Chevrolet and bought it for cash. This was in 1953 so it was pretty old but it was new to me. Now I had my own transportation to and from school, to and from work at the drive-inn, and was able to run errands for mom and dad and take them places they wanted to go when I was available. Dad actually helped me buy the required insurance from Royal Cox Agency in Elkin.

About this time Charlie left the drive-inn for other employment and the new manager gave me the additional responsibility of putting out placards in windows of businesses advertising the coming attractions for free passes. I got paid extra for that and still was the projectionist so for the time and my age, I was doing pretty good financially.

Now that I had a car, had a little cash, and cleaned up my hygiene habits, I was ready to talk to the girls. Seems like most of the ones I approached still remembered me as the snotty nose, rusty ears, dirty kid that I was earlier in life but I had changed. There were a few that agreed to ride with me in my car, go to the movies with me, and maybe have a hot dog at Ed Church's drive-inn. But, I didn't have a lot of time to spend with these people either.

Directly across Highway 67 from the drive-inn was a house where a lady lived with her two daughters and one small son. The youngest daughter was about my age. On occasions she would cross the highway and bring her little brother with her to the drive-inn. They would sit on the outdoor benches and watch the movie. They were never charged and they seldom stayed for the full feature. Her name was Peggy. I would chat with them during their visits and began getting real friendly with Peggy. She was a tiny thing and really cute as she could be. Sometimes she would come over and sit with me until closing and I would take her home. Since both of us were still in school and I worked every night, the only time we could really get together was Saturday and Sunday but I had to be at work at 6PM. This relationship was no puppy love like back when I was 8-10 years old. She was real and I liked her very much. We dated as we could, drove up to the mountains, and just being together was all that mattered.

Charlie had now left and some of the other regulars had left employment at the drive-inn. Business was going downhill and it was sold. The new owners wanted to start running X-rated movies so I began feeling out positions in one of the three theaters in downtown Elkin. They were going to have an open projectionist position at the Reeves and I jumped on it and they hired me for that position. Now I was going to school until noon, worked at the Reeves Theater from 1-5PM and back at 7-11PM. This didn't leave much time for study or Peggy now and she had no transportation to visit me at the theater in town. I really liked her a lot and I think she kind of liked me but this arrangement provided too much separation and she found someone else and later married him.

It obviously was not in God's plan for me to have Peggy because not long afterwards is when I met Faye and she was in God's plan for sure.

Melvin McBride, a cousin to the McBride's that lived across from us on Owl Hill, was a fairly close friend of mine and the week the carnival was in town he and I took it all in spending about every dime we had on us. It was then we met Shirley Renegar and Faye Wilmoth also at the carnival brought there by Shirley's dad. I didn't know Shirley but I had seen Faye at school but never had spoken to her. Melvin and I introduced ourselves and we sat down with them at the bingo table. We didn't have enough money to even play bingo.

Sitting there, I looked down at my feet and, would you believe, there lay a five dollar bill. I reached down and picked it up and said where you all want to go, we got money. We got permission from Mr. Renegar to take them for a ride and would bring them home early. We put $1.00 worth of gas in Melvin's old Oldsmobile and went for a hot dog and a Pepsi. We kept our promise, we got them home early and they lived almost next door to each other. I was on cloud nine after that. I fell head over heels for Faye and absolutely could not get over it. I had to see her again and hopefully could handle it myself without the help of Melvin and Shirley. I went to her house and invited her to go out for a ride and she accepted and from then on I was hooked and could not let her go. I visited often, and I became close friends with her mom and dad and we decided we were in love.

Still in high school and in love I decided I would quit school and get a better job and we would get married but Faye discouraged that and I took her advice. She was two years older, had graduated, and I still had my senior year in school. We decided to get married anyway since her parents agreed we could live with them until I could finish school. No way I would to take her to my parents to live with my dad's drinking and abuse.

On Good Friday, April 16, 1954, Faye Wilmoth and I became husband and wife. Preacher Eli Jordan did the honors and my first cousin, Dub, was my best man. Shirley was the maid of honor and no one else attended. We spent our first night together at the Rock Hotel at the top of the mountain in Sparta, North Carolina. We then lived with Faye's parents until I finished school and were able to get out on our own. At one point in time Faye's brother, R. D., had married Cora Alexander and they were spending time with Faye's parents too. Cora was also still in school like I was and we actually had some classes together. On one particular morning Cora decided she wasn't going to school but I went on ahead. During the class that we had together they were calling the roll and when the teacher got to Cora's name, I spoke up and said she was in bed when I left. That got the attention of the class because they didn't know we were living in the same house but with different spouses. I turned a little red and had to explain that remark.

Melvin also married Shirley some time later but it failed even after them having a baby together. Melvin later died from an unknown ailment.

As promised, I continued school and finished the 12th grade and continued working at the theater. After her graduation, Faye worked at a Ben Franklin Store so we were both in love and very happy. I wrote Faye a lot of poems telling her how much I loved her and how my feelings were for her. I also started writing other poems for situations that happened and gave me the incentive to write. I actually had some published in books of poems but they were mostly all vantage press deals with no royalties paid.

With my poetic ability I got up enough nerve to ask one of the most popular girls in the class to nominate me as class poet and gave her a sample of my work She did a good job and I was elected class poet of our graduating class. This is the poem that was published in our high school senior year book.

GRADUATION

Knowledge comes but wisdom lingers,
Opportunity knocks, waves its fingers,
Bidding us to come ahead, and
Leave EHS as one leaves bed.

The golden days here we spent,
Have all, just passed us by.
But when we think of the fun we had,
We all begin to sigh.

Graduation comes but once a year,
It has come again we trust.
We bequeath the things we love so dear,
And part from you we must.

Opportunity knocks but once they say,
For the ones who struggle through.
Knowledge comes but wisdom lingers,
And the class of '55 bid you adieu.

After graduation, we drove to Winston-Salem for me to seek a real job in the real world so we could move out and support each other financially and have our own place to live. This was in 1955 and the response I would get from places like Western Electric, Reynolds, McLean, Hanes, and etc., those returning from the Korean War were being given priority and suggested I volunteer for the military and complete my military "obligation" and it would be easier to find employment afterwards with that behind me.

Faye and I discussed that and we decided together that I would volunteer for the Air Force. Charlie was married and had already joined the Air Force and Faye's brother, R. D., was in the Air Force so on October 3, 1955, I joined the United States Air Force and left for basic training in San Antonio, Texas.

Chapter 12

UNITED STATES AIR FORCE

My four years in the United States Air Force were just like a public job. I worked eight hours and went home. My tour was after the Korean Conflict and before the Vietnam War so it was all considered peace time.

I boarded a Greyhound bus and headed to Charlotte, North Carolina, along with three others from Elkin and several others that I didn't know to be sworn in. They put us up in one of the old downtown hotels and gave us meal tickets to eat at White Castle Restaurant up the street. The next day the swearing in took place and the third day we were on a plane headed to San Antonio, Texas. I had the three months basic training and missed Faye very much. The Air Force also pulled the four teeth that Dr. Fox told me years earlier that I would be losing. Basic training to me was tough but I went in thinking it would be the worst and tried to make the best of it. Being married got me no favors at all. I was still 17 going on 18 just like most of the others. Only one exercise worried me somewhat and that was hand walking a tight rope across a pond of water. You see, I can't swim. If I fell into that pond somebody would have to come after me or I would just drown right there. The guy going in front of me let go and fell into the water, and that rope tightened up like a spring and jerked me several feet into the air but I hung on. It nearly pulled my arms out their sockets but I didn't get wet. We were all carrying half backpacks at the time that that included a shovel, mess kit, canteen, helmet, and half a tent. Your partner carried the other tent half.

I graduated without any bones broken or drowning and received my first assignment. My test scores showed high in hand to eye coordination, whatever that meant, and was assigned to Francis E. Warren Air Force Base in Cheyenne, Wyoming, teletype communications school. My travel allowance was to pay for travel from San Antonio to Cheyenne. I am from North Carolina and that was way out of the way. I decided to go for it anyway and requested an advance two week leave to go home and would worry about how I would get to Cheyenne later. They had informed me I would be going to school and not be at Francis E. Warren AFB very long so they told me it would not be advisable to take Faye.

After my visit with Faye, I boarded a train in Salisbury, North Carolina, and headed for Wyoming. It took several days on the train and it seems like I could walk as fast as it was traveling until it hit the Midwest. It flew then. When I arrived at F. E. Warren AFB, I learned there were several weeks backlog for students to begin school and I would be there probably four to five months for the six weeks of classes. Hey, that was not what I was told. I wanted another two weeks leave and I was going home and bringing Faye back with me. I did just that. I boarded another train and headed east. Soon as I got back home we packed the 1952 Ford I had left with Faye and we headed back to Wyoming. This was just a few days after Christmas and the weather was fine in North Carolina. It was fine when I left Cheyenne. But by the time we crossed the Great Smoky Mountains, we ran into snow and drove in snow and ice from Tennessee all the way to Cheyenne. It seems like we never saw the ground in Cheyenne for three months. Talk about being cold, some days it would be -24 degrees and wind blowing thirty to forty miles per hour. I worked in the base bakery delivering bakery items, bread and cakes and pies to the chow halls and went home every night. Finally, I started to school and it was also eight to five. I was at home at night with Faye.

My next assignment was to Scott Air Force Base in Belleville, Illinois. This was an advanced teletype cryptographer school. We packed up the old 1952 Ford again on Mother's Day with snow on the ground and headed to Illinois. We were still wearing the blue woolies in Wyoming and upon arrival in Illinois it must have been ninety degrees and humidity the same. We came out of our woolies in a hurry. That was one hot, humid place. I believe I preferred the snow, wind, and ice of Wyoming. There was no backlog of students at Scott AFB so I started to school almost immediately. This was also an eight to five job and I was home with Faye at night and weekends.

When we finished this school our next order was for Shiroi Air Force Base in Japan. With only two stripes, A/2C, I didn't qualify for base housing in Japan and was not qualified to take dependents so this was a real big disappointment. In the Air Force less than a year and I would be heading to Japan alone. My brother, Charlie, spent over twenty years in the Air Force and never went across the Atlantic or Pacific.

I made arrangements again to come home before deploying to Japan so Faye could stay with her parents in Elkin for the projected 18 months I would be gone. We sold and gave away most of the things we had accumulated for the apartment and drove our old 52 Ford back home.

It was a very difficult time for me to leave Faye but living with her parents I knew she would be safe and secure during my absence. So, I flew to Oakland, California, and waited for my group to travel to Japan. Several in my group were scheduled to go by ship which would take about 14 days at sea. I dreaded the thought of being at sea for two weeks. I didn't like the water anyway, was subject to motion sickness, couldn't swim, and had no desire for a boat ride. Again, luck was on my side and was scheduled to fly aboard Flying Tiger Airlines. The scary thing about it, though, was, a Flying Tiger airliner made a controlled landing in the pacific while I was waiting for my scheduled flight. The navy had put down a foam runway in the ocean for the airliner to hit and everyone aboard was saved. The rescue teams appeared to be just waiting for the plane to ditch. It was something for me to think about when I boarded my flight to take the same route.

Our flight left Oakland, California, and the first stop was Wake Island. This was for refueling the plane and a rest stop for its crew and passengers. We were allowed to deplane but we were not allowed to leave the terminal building. This was in 1956 and it had not been that long since Wake Island had been a war zone and they told us lots of unexploded arsenal was still scattered all over the island. The runway at Wake Island is almost the total length of the island. Not a very big place but a strategic one. Next stop was Hickam Air Force Base in Honolulu, Hawaii, for a brief layover. One thing I noticed outstanding at Hickam, which was also the Honolulu International Airport, all the civilians getting off the plane had a lei placed around their neck except the ones like us in uniform. We didn't get one.

Then it was on to Tokyo International Airport in Tokyo, Japan. From there we were bused to Shiroi Air Force Base which was about twelve miles north of Tokyo. You take R Avenue out of Tokyo, go to Ueno, then the Matsudo, then to Mutsami, then to Shiroi AFB. We learned fast that you take the base bus to Mutsami and catch the train into Tokyo so it was very convenient for us on our days off if you had the money to enjoy it. On one occasion the brass offered seats to us as volunteers to fly to Taipei, Taiwan, on a junket type trip. All we needed was twenty dollars to cover overnight accommodations and meals. One of the pilots was my commanding officer and I was one of five selected for the trip. First, I got motion sickness early in the flight. Second, the six bunks aboard the plane were for officers only. I had to tough it out. Upon our arrival we were picked up by jeeps for the brass and huge open bed trucks for us, the volunteers. They took us within hearing distance of the heavy artillery of the war that was still going on between Taiwan and China. Maybe I should have gotten a medal for that. The hotel accommodations were one hundred percent tropical. Open air buildings and the open bay sleeping area had mosquito nets hanging above each bed so when you tucked in, you pulled the string and the net spread out above the bed suspended from the ceiling. Believe me, we all used them. The only purpose for this trip as I could tell was to pick up fresh fruit for our base at Shiroi. I saw no other evidence, business conducted or shared secrets, but after all I was a volunteer, filling a vacant seat, what do I know. We did enjoy the local fruits, though, they fed us well.

My time in Japan went pretty fast and like other places where I had been stationed, worked eight hours a day and rest of the time off but shift work was involved so after a complete rotation of shifts you had three days off at one time. I didn't have to pull any KP or any of that kind of stuff because all that was done by the Japanese locals. We had house boys to clean our rooms, shine our shoes, do our laundry, and anything else we needed them for at hardly any out of pocket expense. So, it was pretty soft duty you might say. During my tour in Japan I met my first cousin, Jim Sloop, who was in the Navy and his ship had docked at a nearby port. We went to the USO and had a hamburger. It was the only place in Japan you could get a hamburger. We visited the Pagoda Village like tourists and took in a theater live musical and guess what, they were topless. I also met another friend from Elkin that I graduated from high school with who was also in the Navy. His ship was also docked nearby. We did about the same thing Jim and I did, the USO being our first stop.

I managed to make one enemy in Japan. In our operations center there was one section that only one person on a shift operated on a normal basis. It intrigued me to no end and I wanted to know how and what it was all about. My shift officer approved of training me to operate this equipment and I tried to learn it backward and forward to know all about it that I possibly could. The officers on shifts had no idea of its working capabilities either and after seeing me take it over, they wanted to get some initial training themselves so they would know if it was working or not working depending on who was working that shift. I put together a little training session and mostly officers attended.

As a result of this move, I was promoted to A1/C even though I was twelve or fifteen down on the list. They called this EWQ, or exceptionally well qualified. The enemy I made was next on the list for promotion and he didn't make it. I got his stripe. He wasn't too happy about it either. One night after he had a few drinks too many at the Airmen's Club he came into my room and turned my bunk upside down with me in it. My roommate, a six foot three Indian from Oklahoma, didn't like the commotion that woke him up and grabbed this guy by the throat and hit him so hard he slid several feet down the waxed hallway floor. He also sported a nice cut on his cheek. He never physically confronted me again but every chance he got he had something smart to say. He rotated back to the states never getting over it and never getting promoted before he left Japan.

The 18 months and five days did pass pretty fast and I was glad it was over and headed back home. My next assignment was back to Texas but this time it would be Kelly Air Force Base. Again, travel pay was to Texas and Elkin, North Carolina. It was a long ways out of the way and I had to foot the bill again. It was worth it because after a brief visit in Elkin, Faye and I were together again and headed back to San Antonio, Texas. Shirley actually went with us to Texas after I casually invited her to go as a figure of speech to my surprise. Now I would have to rent a two bedroom apartment and support her as well. May not be easy but we made the offer and she took us up on it. Fortunately, she did go to work at the Baptist Hospital in San Antonio shortly after we arrived but she never contributed to the apartment in any financial way. She stayed until Faye's mom and dad rode the bus from North Carolina to Texas for a visit with us. When they went back to North Carolina, Shirley went with them.

While I was in Japan, the 1957 Ford Fairlane 500 was advertised in a magazine that was in our barracks. I really thought that was the car for me and cut the picture of it out and put it on the front of my locker. One of the first things I did before we left for Texas was trade my 1952 Ford for a solid black 1957 Ford with the gold trim side molding. It was really sharp.

Since there were three of us in the car, we didn't have a lot of room for the things we thought we would need for an apartment so I went looking for a utility trailer to pull behind by new 1957 Ford. There were a lot of trailers but they were too expensive until I found this one wheel swivel type that attached to the rear bumper in two places in lieu of a tongue with a trailer hitch. We loaded everything we had then some in it and took off. We were making good time and doing well until we approached Mobile, Alabama, where there was an eight mile divided highway with several sections of bridges across the wetlands. Shortly after entering this stretch of highway, would you know it, the tire on that one wheel trailer blew out. We had no spare for it and were a long way from anything, especially commercial. A tractor trailer rig stopped and offered his help. After he saw there was nothing he could do, he offered me a ride to the end of the divided highway where there was a service station and maybe I could get help there. Well, I left Faye and Shirley in the car on the side of the road with a flat tire on the trailer and went with the trucker.

At the service station the mechanic told me he could get me a tire from Sears in Mobile but would it would take a while, maybe the next day before he could take care of it. However, he did rent U-haul Trailers, and suggested I rent one of them and he would deliver it to where we were broke down. That sounded like the best deal so we agreed with him. When he saw what we had, he and I actually lifted my little one wheel trailer onto the U-haul and he brought the clamp on hitches, hooked us up, and away we went, back on our way to Texas.

Another incident occurred when we stopped for gas at a gas station somewhere along the way in a kind of isolated area. While I was pumping the gas, Shirley began flirting with two young boys, teens, standing on the curb in front of the station. They appeared to be taking the flirting seriously and I started to get a little anxious about what they were up to. I rushed into the station and paid for the gas and when I returned to my car, the two teens were leaning up against the car talking to Shirley and Faye and appeared to be trying to get in the car. This was a little scary and I rushed to start the car and put it in gear and began pulling away. The two teens were trying to keep up with me yelling, hey don't run off with my girls. I didn't know if they were going to give us a chase or what but fortunately they did not follow and was I relieved. We had a few words about this going down the road and it was not to happen again.

We arrived in San Antonio without further incident, tired, but glad to be where we more than likely would be stationed for the remainder of my Air Force tour of duty. Kelly AFB was kind of on the other side of town from Lackland AFB where I spent my basic training and had big airplane tankers and lots of jets headquartered there. This place had lots of brass and a lot going on. I went right to work and, again, it was eight to five like public work except you rotated shifts. I worked three days on day shift, off a day, three days on evening shift, off a day, three days on midnight, off three days. Not a bad rotation but getting used to working all shifts took some getting the hang of when to sleep and when not to sleep. My supervisor was a Warrant Officer and, would you believe it, he was from Bethania, North Carolina, a suburb of Winston-Salem. He and I got along well and actually teamed up in a car pool. I liked Kelly AFB and thought about re-enlisting for another four or six years but had second thoughts after I lost out on special duty to Canada. I had an opportunity to transfer to Embassy Duty in Canada, France, or Germany. This job would permit wearing civilian clothes and work in the United States Embassy Building. I volunteered for Canada but seniority beat me out of it so France and Germany were not as appealing as Canada and I left the Air Force after my four years enlistment was completed. You wouldn't believe how stupid I was. Remember that one wheel trailer I pulled from North Carolina to Texas. Well, leaving Texas I did the dumbest thing. I bought another one wheel swivel trailer. This time I went to Sears and bought a spare tire and tube just in case. Fortunately, I didn't need it this time. Sears actually took the tire and tube back and gave me a refund in North Carolina. Couldn't beat Sears during that time.

At this time, Charlie was still in the Air Force and he and Nell were stationed in Canada. He rotated back to the United States and, believe it or not, he was transferred to Kelly Air Force Base and took the same desk I had just vacated when I was discharged. We came that close to crossing paths in the Air Force but not quite.

Sam had now married Shirley Cranford from Elkin and had also joined the Air Force and was stationed at Pope Air Force Base in North Carolina. He and Shirley were living in Spring Lake, North Carolina. He never had a permanent transfer overseas but did temporary duty in Vietnam. So, all three of us boys had United States Air Force careers, mine and Sam's four years each and Charlie in excess of twenty years.

Chapter 13
Finding a Job

My first order of the day arriving back in Elkin after my four year stint in the United States Air Force was finding work. With a car payment and rent in San Antonio, we were not able to save much money at all. Matter of fact we saw times we had to hock my watch to get enough gas to get to and from the base. I always paid it off and got my watch back on payday. Faye and I moved back in with her mom and dad temporarily until we could find a job and get on with our lives.

Dad told me his supervisor said for me to come on down to Chatham's he had a job for me anytime. That was actually the last place I wanted to work because Elkin being a one horse town and Chatham's was the horse. The only people in Elkin that were in the middle class were the doctors and lawyers. The rest were Chatham relatives or lower class wage earners. My best bet was to return to Winston-Salem and start over like I had done exactly four years earlier to no avail.

Western Electric was my first choice as I arrived in Winston-Salem to begin the ultimate task. Before, the story was it was all they could do to hire those coming home from Korea. Now it was different. I completed an application and was interviewed and sure enough I had an offer of real employment with Western Electric.

Since I was a communication trained specialist now, I had potential. The offer turned out to be located on Kwajelein Island, located in the Pacific Ocean. No dependents were allowed and it would be working with the Nike/Zeus missile program. It was a three year rotation back to the U.S. It didn't take long to decline this offer. I told them I wanted to work in this building here at 3300 Lexington Road but sorry nothing available here at this time.

My next stop was McLean Trucking Company on Waughtown Street. I thought I could be a dispatcher or something like that. I had always wanted to drive a big rig but after getting married I didn't think that would work. After filling out an application at McLean, I also got an offer for employment. They said they were in need of drivers badly and they would train at their expense and put me on the payroll at the same time. I had to decline this one, too. I just couldn't take a job "yet" driving a truck long haul across the United States.

The third stop all in the same day, I went to R. J. Reynolds Tobacco Co., which was the largest employer in Winston-Salem at the time. Sure enough, after completing the application and interview I was offered a sales position in Atlanta. Now that wouldn't have been bad and years later I regretted turning that position down. But no, I wanted to work in the Reynolds Building, 401 North Main Street. Sorry, they said, nothing available at this time but if I didn't like Atlanta how about Illinois. I said no thanks and left the Reynolds Building.

At this time, R. J. Reynolds had tenants in the Reynolds Building, insurance agents, railroad offices, stock market offices, doctors offices, and Western Union Telegraph Company. Western Union was two doors down from the main entrance to the Reynolds Building and I said what the heck, I think I will go in here and see if any of the

84

Western Union equipment was anything like what I had operated in the Air Force. To my surprise most of the equipment, maybe a little older, I was very familiar with. The teletype machines were, the tape cutters all were what I had seen and operated. I could read punched tape and could type about 100 words a minute on a teletype writer. I never thought about Western Union being on my list until now.

I asked for the manager and was introduced to Mr. Leon Milhous, who was the manager, and also to the District Manager who had a desk in this office and was responsible for four states, North Carolina, Virginia, West Virginia, and Maryland. I explained to both of them that I just got out of the Air Force and was very familiar with all the equipment they were using, could read tape, and was a very fast typist. Their response was a blessing. The night manager had been drafted into the army and they were looking for someone with teletype experience to replace him. I was their man and I was hired on the spot.

Western Union was unionized and the Winston-Salem office had 12 employees. I was asked to go to work immediately to begin training routines and reported back the very next day. The position of night manager was posted for the union employees to bid on but they felt like there would be no bids for the 3:30PM-12 midnight position. I was wrong. Mrs. Shirley Rufty bid on the job and was awarded the position of night manager. That left her position open which was 1:30-10PM so I was reduced in title but still got the night differential pay and accepted. Shortly after Mrs. Rufty was awarded that position, she took another position closer to her home in Salisbury, North Carolina, and I got the job of night manager after all.

We continued to live in Elkin for a while and I commuted back and forth to Winston-Salem every day. Faye was working at a Ben Franklin Store and we were doing pretty well financially but the 38 miles one way to Winston-Salem was getting old and we needed to move to Winston-Salem. We started out in an upstairs apartment on South Main Street but later bought a huge mobile home and rented a space for it at O. C. Jolly Trailer Park, located on Highway 67. This went on for almost 6 years when one day the Manager, Leon Milhous, announced his retirement. There had been only three managers I know of in the history of this office and all three had retired as old men.

Mr. Milhous took me to the Bobbitt's Drug Store coffee shop to tell me about his plans and went on to say the District Manager wanted me to take over as non-union Manager of the Winston-Salem Western Union Office. I was shocked and delighted to no end. I was going to be manager and would be there till the day I retired as an old man like the other three. This was real security we hadn't really had since we were married, so after being married for almost 10 years we started our family.

Chapter 14
Kids at Last

Our decision to start a family didn't take long to come to pass. Faye was pregnant in no time. We still lived in Winston-Salem but still went to our family doctor in Elkin. He was Dr. Claude McNeil and Faye said up front she wanted Dr. McNeil to be the one who would take care of her during the pregnancy and deliver our first child. That was fine because Elkin was only about 36 miles from our house straight up Highway 67. Near term we could stay at her parents in order to be really close to the hospital in Elkin if it came down to that and if we so desired. So, we had a plan and the months flew by without incident or any problems.

Getting near time to go, Faye began to have contractions and we jumped in the car and headed to Elkin Hospital. It was a false alarm and they sent us home. After that we decided it might be best if we stayed with her mom and dad since this was our first child and we didn't really know what to expect, especially now that we have had a false alarm.

The contractions came again shortly after that and we were glad to be in Elkin at the time. She was admitted to the hospital this time and then the wait began. They then told us that Dr. McNeil was out of town and would not be the one to deliver our first child. Actually it would be Dr. Hal Stewart, and Faye had graduated from high school with him. That was a little difficult to accept but we knew Dr. Stewart and liked him very much so it was not a problem, just a disappointment.

The wait grew long and it wasn't because of any problems, it was because we just got there a little early and they didn't want to send us back home again. During this time period hospitals would not allow anyone in the delivery room except the expectant mother. The father and any family present would have to wait in the waiting room until the doctor came and told you the news. In my case, neither one of my parents or Faye's parents were with us. In fact, no family members were present but the two of us. She was in the delivery room and I was in the waiting room.

During the hours that passed I wrote another poem especially for the time at hand.

MY LITTLE BOY #1

I wish someone else could see,
My little boy, here next to me.
You would say, he's so dear,
And I would say he's always near.

He is such a sweet little doll,
And never does he cry at all.
His hair is red, like his dad,
He's never angry, never sad.

You can't see him, but I can,
Every time he moves his little hand.
You can't tell when he's near,
But I can, he's beside me here.

He doesn't have a name as yet,
Someday he will though, you bet.
He only lives in behind,
His grateful fathers mind.

Finally Dr. Stewart came out of delivery and to the waiting room where I was patiently waiting and announced the good news. It's a boy and everybody was doing just fine. After another wait that seemed like eternity I finally got to see Faye and our little boy. It was a happy moment in our lives and a very special moment at that. We both agreed to name him Todd Harold Hinson. He was born on March 24, 1964.

Our family plan was not complete, however, and we planned just as soon as Todd was out of diapers and Faye had regained her stamina we would go for a second child. We didn't really want Todd to be an only child, had seen some things about that we didn't like. After a couple years we decided we were ready. I still had the manager job at Western Union and Faye didn't have to work any more.

Time flies when you are having fun. Faye was pregnant again in no time and this time we kind of knew what we were doing. We were now experienced at this. We again placed our trust in Dr. McNeil in Elkin to take care of her and the pregnancy and would commute from Winston-Salem to Elkin as necessary and when the time comes, we could again spend some time at her parent's house to be close to the hospital. Everything moved absolutely smooth as silk and when the contractions were where we thought they should be we proceeded to Elkin Hospital. It was time, and Scott Duane Hinson was born on April 22, 1967.

I wrote another poem while I was waiting for our second child. This is how it goes.

MY LITTLE BOY #2

This is the story of yearning for love.
So great a desire it shone from above.
Yet so great and powerful it may be,
It still doesn't happen or exist you see.

Now my little boy, the image of me,
Has auburn hair, greenish eyes you see.
Rosy little face, round full and firm,
And talks, his tongue wiggles like a worm.

He plays all day and minds his dad,
He never cries, unhappy or ever sad.
And every day as I leave the house,
He's right beside me still as a mouse.

He's always happy, his father is glad,
But, he has yet a mother which is so sad.
He hasn't been born from a woman so kind,
He just lives in his fathers mind.

This completed our plan but now the mobile home we had been in for quite some time was getting awfully small with two kids. I still thought of the security I had with Western Union and we decided to go for a house. We had been looking at a new house in the Oldtown section of Winston-Salem for a month or so and decided to go for it. The price of the house with three bedrooms, two baths, living room, den and kitchen combination, carport and sundeck was for us. It had been on the market a while but it was a new house, no one had ever lived in it and it had never been deeded. The price was $19,900. This was 1969, don't forget, so we purchased it and still live in it 40 years later.

Chapter 15
Our Two Boys

Mom and dad had three boys, Charlie, me, and Sam. In keeping with the namesake, it was odd that the three of us had two boys each, no girls. Charlie and Nell had Mike and Steve and they have lived most of their lives in Alaska. Sam and Shirley had Derrick and Kevin and they have lived most of their lives in Winston-Salem, North Carolina. Faye and I had Todd and Scott. Most of their lives have been in the Winston-Salem area. Todd and his wife, Dana, live in the Clemmons area. Scott and his wife, Lisa, live in the King area. Both are close enough to visit often.

Our two boys were raised in an atmosphere that we thought would take them into the world clean and wholesome and let them decide where it would take them as adults. Working as I was early in their lives, it was nights and weekends and seldom did we take them to church. Then later on I was doing so much traveling all I wanted to do was to be with my family and do family things together. My feelings on religion were and still are that I am a strong believer in God and I think the bible is my guide to life. I went to church as a kid and that is where I got my strength to lead my life as I have. I think the church is good for you but I also think that some people in the church that I grew up in were there for the show and not for the salvation of God. For instance, on occasions when I was commuting from Elkin to Winston-Salem to my job at Western Union I was asked on numerous occasions by some noted church leaders in Elkin to stop by the ABC store and bring them back a fifth of their favorite liquor since Elkin did not have an ABC store and they would pay me to do this. It was all legal since I could purchase up to five fifths and transport as long as the seals were not broken. But, this is one of the reasons my going to church went to the back burner. I did not drink and I did this as a favor but they went to church on Sunday as if they were good and wholesome and I pictured them as hypocrites. I guess I was one also.

After we moved to Winston-Salem we found about the same thing with some of the people we knew that were faithful church attendees. Another thing, we were just getting started out in the business world and it seemed everyone else was so much higher in society, in business status, and overall better than us. We lived in a house trailer. We didn't know anyone that attended church that lived in a house trailer. This also had an effect on our decision about going to church. I think the word to describe our status is we were intimidated. But, if children were not welcome at places we did not visit those places with or without them. On occasions we did go back to Elkin and attend East Elkin Baptist Church where I was baptized. We also attended once in a while with some of our closest friends at their church when they made a specific invitation. Todd and Scott probably were too young to remember many, if any, of these visits. So, it was our decision and deliberate decision to let them go in the direction that their beliefs led them by providing an environment conducive to their beliefs and it worked. They were not trained to believe this or believe that as a child but they were trained right from wrong in the sense the bible teaches. We are proud of our two boys and love them very much for the direction they took.

Todd and Scott got along very well growing up. They didn't have the new electronic technology we have today but they made use of what they did have and it was the latest at the time. If we couldn't afford certain things they wanted somehow they got them either from our sacrifice or Faye's mom who pampered them. We visited Six Flags Theme Park in Virginia, Six Flags in Ohio, and Six Flags in Georgia. We took them to the beach and to the mountains. We took them to Disney World in Florida just after it first opened. We visited the tourist attractions all through Florida. So, they didn't miss any of that. They just didn't have that DVD, Game Boy, and etc. They just were not available in the 60's and early 70's. They did get a trip of a lifetime to Alaska when we drove up to deliver the Lincoln which Charlie bought in Winston-Salem during his visit when Sam died. The overnight trip to Valdez via the glaciers and Prince William Sound was pretty exciting for them as well as the flight back, which was their first flight. That was pretty exciting for them too.

The trip to Alaska was Todd's senior year in high school and he had decided to pursue a career in computer science. Again, we did not direct, suggest or insist this or that career or college. He made his own decisions and we complied with all the help we could provide him. He ranked second in his high school senior class which was a pretty significant achievement He decided to attend Western Carolina University for the computer program they offered based on his research and we agreed. I didn't know where the money was going to come from but I did not hesitate to support his decision. He was accepted and we managed to get the first semester paid and away he went.

Faye and I and Scott took Todd to WCU and got him checked in. First thing we noticed was a trash barrel at each entrance of the dorms. We spent the night in one of the dorms and the next day those barrels at the entrances were running over with beer cans. Well, what have we got into here? It was party time and Todd had never been exposed to "party time." In any event, he stayed, we left and came back home. We had helped him get his first car and when he came home, we allowed him to take his car back so he could come home whenever he had time and wanted to. His first problem, his assigned roommate was a party animal and returned to the room late at night and always under the influence. Todd was there to study and he did. He made the Dean's List the first semester but the roommate had soured his interest in continuing after the first semester and he wanted to come home so we agreed for him to come home. We talked to his high school guidance counselor about this at a later date and she blamed us for not introducing him to the "real world".

Todd has since graduated from High Point University with a degree and is gainfully employed in computer technology and a leader in his church. He was hired temporarily to preach when their full time preacher left their church and he often fills in for the current preacher when he needs to be somewhere else on occasion. He and Dana have two adopted children, Andrew and Emily. Todd and Andrew have also been to Nicaragua where they were on a Church of Christ mission trip.

On the other hand, Scott was not interested in going to college and he immediately went to work after graduating from high school. He also studied computer science and has followed that as his career.

Scott worked as a computer programmer for a small company that did mostly automobile insurance and financial documents. He moved from this job to Piedmont Airlines, later becoming USAIR. This experience gave him the knowledge to proceed in this career field and fortunately he needed it as the company was carved up and moved out of Winston-Salem. He was able to move on to a local insurance company and remains at this company in Winston-Salem. As fate would have it, though, he was let go for several months before being rehired as a contractor. During that time he worked with an independent company that has programmers offshore and worked as go between and visited the offshore location in Romania. This company was trying to grow and just couldn't get to the point where he could continue to afford Scott. Again, he was rehired at the insurance underwriter as a contractor hoping to get rehired as a permanent soon.

Scott has also followed his own mind in what he wants to do and where he wants to worship and is a leader in his church. He teaches Sunday school classes at church and is involved in most of the church's activities. He likes to help the disadvantaged and has been to the flood ravaged area in the western North Carolina Mountains with help to those people in need. He has been to Mobile, Alabama, after the hurricane Katrina on two occasions and has been on mission trips to El Salvador. Scott met his wife, Lisa, at USAIR after her divorce from her first husband. She already had two boys, Michael and Daniel, and after they were married they had Alyssa. Since this was not enough, Scott and Lisa went to China and adopted a newborn little girl, Kayli, who had been abandoned on the steps of the children's home.

Chapter 16

CHANGING TIMES

Up until this point, Faye and I had provided most of the transportation for my parents and her parents when they wanted to visit some of the family or maybe a trip to the mountains. We occasionally took my parents and Faye's parents together with us to the mountains. Now things were different because we had a family of four and only two more at a time could go with us so we had to be really careful not to upset either of our parents when we took the other one somewhere. We took my parents to Fort Bragg to see Sam and Shirley while he was still in the Air Force and stationed at Pope Air Force Base. We took Faye's parents to Columbia to see Faye's brother, R. D., and his wife, Cora, when he was stationed at Shaw Air Force Base. We visited both her parents and mine often but we had a problem when we visited and my dad was drinking. We would not allow our two boys to be subjected to his condition so that created a problem with us spending more time with Faye's parents than mine.

My dad had now retired from Chatham's and never wanted to leave the house to visit anyone. All he wanted to do was to drink and, as mom put it, give her enough tongue lashing to kill a mule. In September 1965, mom was friends with a lady that was a housekeeper at the Elkin Hotel and she was pregnant. As they talked, her friend suggested she apply for the job she had while she was on maternity leave and get away from some of that tongue lashing. Every time mom went out, it was where you been, who did you see, who did you talk to, and so this sounded like a good idea to at least get away part of the day anyway.

On September 14, 1965, mom went to work at the Elkin Hotel. This was her first job at public work in her lifetime at the age 53. She had talked it over with my dad that one of them needed to get out and do something to make some extra money. Everything was getting so expensive, she needed new glasses, prescriptions they both had to take, groceries, and utilities. Her glasses were round thick outer edge with a thin center circle which by this time was her eyes. She could only see the form of things and could not see the features without them. Mom was considered legally blind by this time.

Charlie and Nell were still in Alaska and would send them a few dollars occasionally as a token since they were so far away they seldom ever came back to visit. So, that Tuesday morning she went to work at eight o'clock and worked until Saturday, twelve o'clock and got paid $15.00. She paid $6.00 she owed on her revolving bank account and $5.00 on her new glasses that cost $50.00. Next payday mom gave dad $10.00 of her check and he used it to buy a rake. He had never raked leaves before but he was now. She also bought him a hot water bottle to help the blood circulation in his feet when he went to bed. She also bought him four pair of socks and he really liked them, she said.

Dad broke his arm on December 10, 1965, helping Cal Griffin feed his pigs while both of them were drunk, of course. So, mom had to quit her job to take care of him because it was his right arm. He said he heard it snap, sounded like a corn stalk cracking. Mom said he changed like a baby, was so sweet and good because he needed her now more than ever. She then decided that she would rather sit at home and watch the soaps and be with dad than to put up with that every time she came home, especially for only $15.00 a week. That was the end of her employment. It was then back to dividing dad's $93.90 social security check to pay all the bills.

Some time after recovering from breaking his arm, dad had a pretty serious heart attack. He was rushed to the hospital and they brought him back with defibrillator shocks. His chest was black and blue from the bruising. He had been saved several years ago and baptized, dedicating his life to the Lord and knew he was now close to death. He had slowed down somewhat on his drinking and actually had been going back to church with mom when transportation was to his liking. He wasn't one to do much asking for a ride now and depending still on mom for those arrangements. While he was in the intensive care unit, I was visiting with him and he started telling me about a vision he had experienced during this heart attack. He said,

"I was at my own funeral. After the service the casket rose into Heaven. When it got there, it stood on its end and I stepped out. I had on my never changing robe. Jesus said, can I help you? I told Him I wanted to go to Heaven. He said you are here. I looked around and He said he can go too. He was talking about Sam. There was two large groups of people and the sky was bright yellow as if it was gold, just like the bible says. I could tell you a lot more but there is some people who wouldn't believe me."

After he was discharged from the hospital and had gone back home, he became confused, incontinent and it was more than mom could handle. We made arrangements for him to be transferred to a nursing home. In no time he didn't know where he was, who we were, or anything about his past, or present. He had completely lost everything except his ability to exist. On one occasion I witnessed them feeding him and they put a spoon full of beef in his mouth. He immediately spit it out and would not eat another bite. He was 99.9% disabled and confused but he still knew the taste of beef which he despised and continued to refuse to eat. On April 30, 1984, he passed away at the age of 85. Mom lived alone in a HUD duplex for a few years after that but she became incompetent and she also was moved to a nursing home. She died December 8, 1997, also at the age of 85.

The position of manager of the Western Union office in Winston-Salem was a non-union position. All the other positions were unionized as I was prior to being appointed to manager. Now my balloon was about to burst, I would not be the manager retiring as an old man as those in the past. Management had decided that this office manager would be put back into the union and they had other plans for me. I was being promoted to Area Manager, the states of North Carolina, Virginia, West Virginia, and Maryland. I would have a company automobile with unlimited personal usage, an American Express expense account and an office in the Winston-Salem WU office and responsible for all the contract agencies that represent Western Union in these four states. There were approximately 500 different locations in 500 different towns including the company operated WU offices. Not only was I responsible for their existence, I was responsible for maintaining their existence meaning if one quit, I would have to replace it based on Federal Communications standards at that time. Three people would report to me to make this happen, Mr. Ken Spivey from Asheville, North Carolina, Mr. Dennis Stacey from Burlington, North Carolina, and Mr. Kenneth Hill from Goldsboro, North Carolina. The change was effective immediately.

As we developed a plan to handle this project, geographically it was great. Spivey would get most of the western areas, Hill would handle the eastern areas, and Stacey and I would work central and go north. It was a huge task to meet all FCC requirements, signage, service, and etc. We worked great together, though, and when one of us was getting behind the other one was used to help get caught up again.

Western Union decided they would close all the company operated offices and convert them to contract agencies and it would be up to us to sign contracts in each town a company operated WU office existed. Now the approximately 500 locations would all be agents and all WU employees would be let go with a liberal severance package depending on their years of service. With the help of the managers of the major WU offices like Raleigh, Charlotte, Richmond, Charleston, and Baltimore, this was accomplished and I still had a job. This required a tremendous amount of travel and all of it had to be by automobile. The little remote towns we covered were not accessible to fly into and the time it would take to fly and drive was about as much time as it would take to drive to start with. I was fortunate to have good people working with me and we were able to be home almost all weekends, usually Monday and usually Friday if we cared to plan it that way. Since we were all four married, we planned it that way most of the time so we could be home with our families. Dennis and I actually took our fishing gear to the coast and fished at night on one trip I recall. We caught 15 sand sharks that night and nothing else off the pier at the Gold Coast Beach pier.

Charlie Thomas had been my replacement as manager at the WU office in Winston-Salem. I had known Charlie for quite some time as a relief manager. During this time, Western Union covered all Wake Forest University basketball and football home games, the NCAA tournaments, and any and all dignitaries' visits to the area. We would provide teletype service and an operator to transmit the stories reporters wrote directly to their newspaper office. Sometimes we would be given more tickets than we needed to staff the affair and, at our discretion, would give them to our friends or whoever rather than not using them at all. Charlie was sharing some of these tickets with R. J. Reynolds Tobacco executives as our largest account and gaining respect and 'points' for the future whether it be intentional or not. In any event, Charlie was eventually offered a position with R. J. Reynolds Tobacco Company and immediately submitted his resignation from Western Union. His resignation ultimately came to me and I was not surprised but his timing was not in his best interest. I had been instructed to close the Winston-Salem Western Union office and convert it to a contract agent and if Charlie left now he would forfeit a severance package that he was not aware of. Otherwise, if he stayed until the office officially closed he would get a severance package which, in his case, was several thousand dollars.

My job was straight forward, but Charlie being a friend of mine, I discouraged him from resigning by denying his resignation without telling him the closing was forthcoming. He obtained permission from RJR to delay his coming aboard in order to remain with Western Union until a "replacement" was found. We proceeded with our objective and in a few weeks issued Charlie's notice that his job was being terminated and presented him with a nice severance payment. He then went to work for R. J. Reynolds Tobacco Company in Winston-Salem. I am not sure Charlie understood my involvement in his termination, but maybe he did. A few years later he came through for me.

As time passed, Federal Communications Commission relaxed some of their rules and regulations for Western Union and I was relieved of West Virginia and Maryland but still covered North Carolina and Virginia. Most of our work now consisted of agency inspections and occasional replacement. Replacement became very difficult and we were finally allowed to de-list some locations where it was practically impossible to find a contract agent. I tried to justify my job and the salary being paid to me and it seemed in the not too distant future I would have worked myself out of a job and would no longer be needed.

In 1977 my office telephone rang and it was Charlie Thomas. He wanted to know if I was interested in going to work for RJR. I had to think for a minute. I had offers 20 years before but not in this building. Charlie said he was getting a promotion to another department and his manager wanted to know if he knew of anyone with the same type background he had, customer service, excellent typist, sales oriented, and administrative experience. If I was interested, his manager wanted to talk to me. Thinking I had almost worked myself out of job at WU, I thought this might be what I needed. I was forty years old and if I was going to make a change I better do it now. I agreed to meet Charlie's manager and arranged for an interview with Mr. John Orr, Manager of Duty Free Sales. John talked with me at length and introduced me to the Director of Duty Free Sales and proceeded to give me a typing test. I apparently met their expectations and was immediately offered the position being vacated by Charlie. They also gave me a five hundred dollar salary increase from my current salary at Western Union. It stunned me for a moment. I had to give Western Union two weeks notice since I had almost 20 years service with WU. So, I accepted the position with the understanding that I would also have to keep my work at Western Union caught up during the two weeks notice but no travel. I submitted my resignation to Western Union and began working at RJR at the same time. My Western Union home office manager was a little upset and asked why I didn't give them a chance to counter offer. They thought that I was not serious but it was serious and a done deal. Thanks to Charlie Thomas I was now working for R. J. Reynolds Tobacco Company and in the same building that I had applied twenty years before. This department was responsible for duty free sales, cigarettes sold in the United States but smoked outside the United States. Those qualified to purchase duty free were U.S./Canadian Border stores, U.S./Mexican Border stores, U.S. International Airports, U.S. Military Ships Afloat, Commercial, foreign flag ships, and U.S. Commercial Fishing Vessels fishing outside the 12 miles limits of the U.S. This consisted of an area completely around the borders of the U.S., plus it included Hawaii, Alaska, and Latin America. This was a big area with approximately 50 sales representatives to cover it. I was the Administrative Assistant to the Department's Sales Manager handling most of the correspondence, price changes, shipping promotional items, and maintaining the customer listings consistent with tax, customs, and other requirements governing duty free sales as well as doing collections from the U.S. Navy ships afloat purchases. This was a pretty cool job with exotic appeal working with several different nationalities and destinations.

Traveling to these areas was an extra bonus in itself. There was no problem with expenses, we were encouraged to stay in the right places. Customer entertainment was expected and usually a must. In my case, I enjoyed NASCAR racing and had the opportunity to entertain our customers at all the big tracks south and east of the Mississippi. If it was golfing, then somebody else got the trip because I didn't play golf, even though I was on most of the biggest and best courses in the United States with my co-workers responsible for the customers playing.

One of the highlights of my second career working for R. J. Reynolds Tobacco Company was when I had the opportunity to go aboard Air Force One during President Reagan's presidential term and getting a grand tour of everything from the President and Mrs. Reagan's suite to the oval conference room, the press room to the galley, including menus and jelly beans, a favorite of President Reagan. Not many civilians can say they have been aboard Air Force One, but I have.

Chapter 17

SECOND CAREER

On January 12, 1982, my younger brother, Sam, died in a single car accident from head trauma. He was only 42 years old, leaving his wife, Shirley, and their two young boys, Derrick and Kevin. My older brother, Charlie, and his wife, Nell, flew from Alaska to North Carolina to be with the family and attend the funeral. I let him have one of my two cars to move about visiting all the relatives and to have free transportation while he was here.

In previous visits Charlie flew from Alaska to Eugene, Oregon, where they build motor homes and on at least two occasions purchased one and drove to North Carolina and other places of interest like Florida where he owned some real estate. Then he would drive it back to Alaska and put it up for sale at Alaska prices but he bought it at Oregon prices. He told me this difference was enough to almost pay for the trip home.

This trip after the funeral he went looking for a car to take back to Alaska to do the same thing, North Carolina price vs. Alaska price to again supplement his expense for the trip home. He purchased a new Ford Thunderbird but he had seen a used Lincoln Versailles he really wanted. That is when he popped the question to me. If he also bought the Lincoln, would Faye and I and our two boys drive it to Alaska when school was out in June. We had never even thought of going to Alaska to visit them and this was an opportunity we probably should go for and we agreed to do it. We had from January until June to plan the trip. Charlie had sent us milepost markers showing where facilities would be and explained that there were still 1000 miles of dirt/gravel road through Canada, the ALCAN Highway, but it would be summertime and we would not have to worry about snow and ice. We were really excited planning the trip and looked forward to the day we would be leaving. I planned two weeks vacation at RJR and got approval so just as soon as school was out for the summer we took off on a journey, and we had no idea what it would be like.

Our trip included a stop in Knoxville, Tennessee, where the world fair was held, on to Chicago, Mount Rushmore, and crossed the border at Sweetgrass, Montana. I have never seen so many deer along the way, in the road, in the median, everywhere. We were lucky we didn't hit one. When we crossed in Canada we got our first experience in currency exchange, which was in our favor at the time. We also were amazed at the number of oil rigs along that paved stretch of highway. Then, all of a sudden the blacktop ended and dirt/gravel began with no warning and I was going about 55 MPH and immediately in front of me was a high pile of gravel in the middle of the road. I hit the brakes hard in order to maneuver around to the right of the pile of gravel as oncoming traffic was coming from the left side. This was a wakeup call for me from that point on because it was definitely dirt/gravel for the next 1000 miles. We saw big horn sheep, obviously wild horses, and more deer. The places we had marked for overnight were no Holiday Inn. Some were hunters' cabins, rail workers' overnight beds, but we did stay in pretty decent places, even though the only light in the room was a bulb burning from a generator at the office. The food available along the way was not like North Carolina's either but we managed well enough to not go hungry for sure. At one point along the ALCAN it had rained and the mud stuck underneath the fenders like snow does until it rubbed the tires. When we would meet a tractor and trailer rig it would be running about 90 MPH, it seemed, and it would splatter you with gravel or mud, whichever the weather happened to be. At one motel we stopped at, I was getting our clothes out of the trunk and noticed a liquid dripping underneath the gas tank. I thought surely it wasn't a ruptured gas tank. I touched the liquid and it didn't smell like gas or oil but more like water. That's when I checked our Styrofoam cooler where we had packed drinks and sandwich meat, and the dirt/gravel road had been so rough on it a hole had worn in the bottom and the melted ice was leaking out. Boy, was I relieved. We did get a lot of nicks in the paint, cracked windshield, and a cracked headlight, but nothing major.

During our visit with Charlie and Nell in Anchorage they had planned a trip for us to take his camper on an overnight trip. This trip was really nice, even though it was about 25 degrees. Our first stop was the Portage Glacier, then to Whittier where we put the camper on a train to Prince William Sound where we put the camper on a ferry and sailed across the Prince William Sound watching sea lions and seals follow us to Valdez, Alaska. We also saw Columbia Glacier. We spent the night in a hotel in Valdez, and then left the next day heading back to Anchorage. This also took us to a huge glacier area where we were able to get out and walk on top of the glaciers ice. This was indeed a trip of a lifetime for us, and really special for our two boys, Todd and Scott.

During our overnight trip to Valdez, I noticed there were a lot of fishing villages that fish in international waters, big supply houses, and canneries along the way. When we got to Valdez there were foreign flag ships taking on oil and U.S. flag ships bringing supplies, automobiles, and everything else to Anchorage since by road would be not only expensive but time consuming. I already knew Anchorage International Airport had a duty free shop. This was the business I was now working with RJR and nobody had been up there to sign up this business which they would be eligible to buy duty/tax free cigarettes. There were Sea-land ships in the area and Sea-land was owned by R. J. Reynolds at that time. I had found a gold mine for our department, we just needed to get a sales representative up there and sign them up to sell our products.

Our trip back to Winston-Salem was the first time Faye and the boys had ever flown in an airplane and we were so anxious our last night in Anchorage we didn't even go to bed. It was June 21st, the longest day of the year, and it never got dark all night long. It was light enough to read a newspaper outside that night. We boarded our flight about 7AM and everyone except me was asleep almost before we got airborne. We had one stop, being Chicago, and we were soon home.

Returning to work, I made it a point to discuss what I had seen in Alaska and suggested that I meet the west coast manager and he and I go to Alaska and see if we couldn't sign a new business for our department. He agreed and in a few weeks after planning we were on our way back to Alaska. This time I was traveling with our west coast manager. We were very successful in signing up suppliers of these fishing vessels and U.S. and Foreign flag ships as well as meeting with the airport duty free shop. This trip was well supported by the new business we achieved for our department at RJR.

This experience advanced my career to work closely with the field sales force and now occasionally I was traveling to all these exotic places. I became responsible for the inventories in the warehouses that supplied these areas and they required inventory checks periodically. I also helped plan most of the sales seminars, selection of a hotel, menu, and recreation each year which we held in the Florida Keys, New Orleans, Miami, New York, and the Tampa area. We always used a first class facility.

The overnight trip to Valdez gave us an experience that after we returned home, we decided we would check out purchasing a motor home. We found it was easier than we thought and bought a used 34 foot Pace Arrow and began using it immediately going to the coast and the mountains. We liked it so well we decided we would trade up for a new Pace Arrow, also 34 foot in length. The new one gave us so much trouble with the exterior walls separating and leaks we were at our wits end. The manufacturer in Pennsylvania picked it up four times for repairs while it was in warranty. They put more miles on it going to and from the factory than we did. After the fourth repair, we traded it for another new 34 foot Pace Arrow, as if we hadn't had enough problems with Pace Arrow, but this one was really nice. I was still working but Faye and I traveled from New York to Florida and west to the Mississippi River. This was how we spent our weekends and our scheduled vacations.

In the meantime, Charlie's cancer of the colon had spread to the liver and the location on the liver made it inoperable, from what I understand. Charlie and Nell's oldest son, Mike, and his wife, Sally, and their two girls, Sarah and Katy, were living in Winston-Salem. They had moved about from Alaska to Winston-Salem more than once but at this time they were in Winston-Salem. Charlie's condition continued to worsen and it appeared the end was eminent and soon.

Mike and his oldest daughter, Sarah, left Winston-Salem and flew to Alaska to be with his dad during this critical time. His wife, Sally, and the younger daughter, Katy, decided they would fly to Florida to visit her parents and then proceed on to Alaska, not knowing how long they would be in Alaska. While Sally and Katy were visiting her parents, they were going shopping with her mom and dad when a tractor and trailer rig reportedly blew a front tire and crossed the median and hit their car head on. Sally, Katy, Sally's mom and Sally's dad were all four killed instantly. Mike and Sarah were in Alaska with his dad on his death bed.

I talked to my boss and made arrangements to do a presentation to Duty Free shoppers at Anchorage International Airport and also visit my brother. I called Charlie and told him I was coming to Alaska to be with them and help in anyway I could. Charlie's response was, we need all the help we can get. Those were his last words spoken to me. By the time I got to Alaska he had gone into a coma and never came out. The doctors told us to talk to him because it was believed some people in a coma can hear but cannot respond even with a smile. I don't know if he knew I was there or not but his youngest son, Steve, and I were the only ones with him when he passed away after midnight.

While in the coma, Charlie had swelled to a point he was not much like he was the last time I saw him. When he passed away, the moisture in his body saturated the sheets around him outlining his body and he returned to his normal size and looks before the coma. Strange.

We had planned this motor home for our retirement but about the time I was getting old enough to retire I began having vertigo problems as well as kidney stones. After retirement we were afraid to go out with the medical condition I was experiencing. Faye was also having extreme pain in her knees and hips from arthritis. Eventually we put it on consignment and didn't try the motor home camping again.

R. J. Reynolds had now begun downsizing and I was nearing the age we could retire if I could get a package. On the second or third round of layoffs I was 57 years old with almost 20 years at RJR and volunteered for a package. The package would take me to 59-1/2, the magic number for no penalties, and both of us could get Social Security at 62, so it worked out great for us. We also were drawing a little pension from the nearly 20 years at Western Union. After four years in the Air Force and nearly 40 years in the work force, we were now retired.

Chapter 18

HEARTACHES AND PAIN

A rthritis had about taken control of Faye's knees and hips and she was in a lot of pain. Our Health Care doctor had prescribed one drug after another in an effort to give her some relief. The one last prescribed and was taken for a considerable period of time was Celebrex. It was one of those drugs that were eventually recalled and afterwards she only took two to four Tylenol a day which was about as good as any prescription drug she had been taking for pain. Over time she had also experienced kidney stones and on the ones that didn't pass lithotripsy was used successfully. In addition she also was diagnosed with spinal stenosis.

In December 1999 her orthopedic surgeon suggested a left knee total replacement would be in order for her condition. We thought the right knee was in worse shape because it had started an inwards bend in the leg and seemed to be more painful than the left one. We elected to go with the total replacement of the left knee and everything went very well. We were able to get home physical therapy and she recovered normally but the right knee was supporting body weight now that the left leg was still healing and causing great pain. In January 2003 we agreed that a total replacement of the right knee was our only hope to relieve the pain. This surgery also went well and she recovered nicely but the pain continued to exist in the right thigh area. We suspected that the replacement of the knee put it back in line with the hip and the hip was radiating pain down the thigh into the right knee. The pain was so intense I took her to the hospital emergency room to see if they could help her get some relief. Their diagnosis was the right hip was damaged by arthritis to the point it needed replaced, the sooner the better.

We consulted our orthopedic surgeon and his x-rays confirmed what the hospital had told us and suggested total right hip replacement before the bone completely gave way. So, in August 2006 she had the right hip totally replaced. They also detected excessive fluid on the brain during a brain scan and in an hours time we were talked into neurosurgery for a brain shunt device. We certainly did not expect that. This was a long healing process but with the help of physical therapists we were able to bring her home for recovery. I noticed she was not quite the same as before but couldn't figure out just what it was. They told me that during the surgery to replace the hip she encountered an erratic heartbeat and after an extremely long period in the recovery room she was taken to the hospital's coronary unit instead of the orthopedic unit for two days. This was a little strange, was it serious, had she fully recovered from the erratic heartbeat, or what was going on. They seemed to shrug it off and said it was no longer a problem, everything was fine. But it wasn't, she was not the same mentally and as time passed she had completely lost her memory how to do anything. She could no longer balance the checkbook that she always had done, she couldn't set the VCR, microwave, clocks, washing machine, dryer, or remember how to cook anything. Then she stopped talking in sentences, only a word or two could be spoken. She stopped watching TV, could no longer read the paper or the magazines subscribed specially for her.

After trying my best to get her to a psychologist, suggested by our family doctor, I finally was able to talk her into going in April 2007. She was diagnosed with Alzheimer's dementia. I questioned the diagnosis to no avail. One doctor said she appeared to be a victim of deprived oxygen, or possibly extreme trauma and not really Alzheimer's dementia. So, we still wonder if the erratic heart condition during surgery was in fact a lack of oxygen or could it have been extreme trauma during the hip replacement surgery. In the past three years I see little change. It doesn't seem she has gotten any worse or any better in her mental capacity or speech ability.

Two years later, in 2008, that hip replacement separated three times, first in February, second in May and third time in September 2008. Each time required ambulance attendants to support lifting her body because of severe pain. After the third separation, the orthopedic surgeon made the call for re-construction to go back in and replace the ball and socket, hopefully not having to replace the parts attached to the bone. This surgery was performed and, fortunately, only a larger ball and socket had to be replaced. After five days in the hospital I brought her home in the car. As we entered the house, I noticed her clothing was getting soaked in blood around the surgical area; and when I started to change the bandage blood squirted from between the stapled incision. I immediately called for an ambulance after being home less than 15 minutes to take her to the emergency room to control the bleeding. Within a couple hours the ER had the bleeding controlled and said we could come home. I stated in certain terms otherwise, she wasn't leaving the hospital until overnight observation to ensure the bleeding was indeed stopped.

They agreed and kept her overnight. I stayed in the room with her all night because we both were really scared seeing that incision bleeding like it was.

We came home from the hospital the next day, which was a Friday. Over the weekend I noticed the bleeding was a lot more than normally it should be so I contacted the doctor for some instructions. They told us to come to the office first thing Monday morning; and in the meantime keep a clean bandage over the incision and if it got increasingly worse take her back to the ER. Well, we survived the weekend and first thing Monday morning we were at the orthopedic surgeon's office. He looked at the incision and called the problem a hematoma. He sent her directly to the hospital for the incision to be reopened and cleaned out and reclosed. This procedure was successful and the bleeding was stopped and after a couple days in the hospital we went back home again.

Faye was progressing very well for someone with two artificial knees and an artificial hip. She was using a walker to steady her walk and we were going out to eat and whatever we normally did, however, she was not getting any better or worse in her memory and ability to make conversation. We learned to communicate with her by asking questions until we got the right question when she indicated she wanted something. She could say yes and no and could repeat any word I would ask her to repeat but she could not say it voluntarily or make a sentence.

Faye was continuing to recover from the neurosurgery for a brain shunt device, hip re-construction, and hematoma at home but still depending on a walker for support. As for the brain shunt device, I am not so sure she needed that procedure but what do you do when a neurosurgeon stands before you and tells you he may be able to bring her back four or five years with this surgery. The previous brain scans either failed to show excessive fluid or the doctors felt it wasn't sufficient to tell us that there was excessive fluid Or maybe they overlooked it, who knows.

We still went out to eat, visit our sons and their families, and tried to provide a normal atmosphere for her. Something new was occurring, though, that we had not experienced before. While sitting on the couch, she threw her head backwards, mouth open and appeared unable to breath. I grabbed her, shook her shoulder and she came out of it. This happened four times that I witnessed and I thought she was having seizures and discussed this with her family doctor.

Then in February 2009 she fell in the kitchen floor and was in severe pain. This fall was apparently caused by what we thought was a seizure. We called the paramedics again and they looked at her and told me they thought her left hip was broken. Wow, that is all we need, she is still recovering from the right hip surgery. The emergency room doctor confirmed what the paramedics told me, the left hip was fractured but not severed. She would require surgery to either repair or replace the left hip. Fortunately, this hip could be repaired with three screws. Downside was it would be three months before she could put body weight on the left leg. While she was in recovery, what we thought was a seizure happened again.

They immediately took her to the intensive care unit and diagnosed the heart had an electrical problem and she would need a pacemaker. It wasn't seizures, it was her heart stopping causing what we thought were seizures. A pacemaker was surgically placed while she was still recovering from the hip surgery. If it could be determined, this was probably what happened in 2006 with the first hip surgery but no doctor will admit, and no lawyer will commit. This further confirms my doubt that a brain shunt device was actually needed. It was the heart causing the falls, not the brain. She now has two implants magnetic controlled, a brain shunt device, a pacemaker, two artificial knees, one hip replacement, and one hip with three screws.

Three months before, body weight on the left leg posed a real problem and now because the right leg was still recovering from the September surgery and would not support her weight. There was no way I could take care of her or handle her with restricted body weight. As bad as we hated to do so, we had to send Faye to a rehab facility for recovery. After 33 days, she was able to get on and off the bed and up and down to a wheelchair. This was good enough for me. I could handle this so we asked the doctor for permission to take her home and she was discharged from the rehab the same day. What am I doing, can I really handle this?

Totally helpless, totally reliable on someone else for moving her, keeping her pain free, hygiene, no control over either bladder or bowels, meeting her appetite needs, it all looked easy at the rehab center. But let me tell you, they are professionals. For me it is a full time job and not always a pleasant one. But one thing is in my favor. She is content, she is happy, she can laugh, she can accept the situation, I believe because I don't think in her mind she knows what the situation really is. So, we manage well and accept the challenge before us.

God knows how much we can handle.

Chapter 19
Alzheimers/Dementia

It is a real accomplishment to reach the seventies in an age with all the turmoil, disease and fast times that we now live in. And to reach that age with a sound mind and body that is not broken is even more of an accomplishment. However, in addition to making the necessary changes in life, another change is slowly taking place. That change is so gradual that you hardly notice it until it is obvious that a change has actually taken place. Obvious meaning is the change of one person is affecting another person, usually a loved one. In order to better understand these changes I have kept a record which is necessary to note what is actually taking place in the mind of the person that this gradual change is taking place. The following are the changes we noticed in my wife, Faye, beginning in 2006.

Faye began experiencing loss of appetite which was the first drastic change noticeable. We thought maybe this was due to all the surgeries she had been through and would recover. She complained about the entire food chain whereby nothing tastes right or good anymore. Food that has always been a mainstay is now too salty, too sweet, or just doesn't taste like it used to. Then there is the idea that it is no longer good for you. Home charcoaled steak is no more, trash the ones in the freezer. Never eat steak at your usual steak places and discourage your spouse to do the same, not good for you. And if you do indulge in these foods you will be accused of eating anything. The bottom line for loss of appetite is, of course, loss of weight and the constant complaining about her food.

Her physical attitude probably came next in a change that appears to be more like depression. This is noted, for example, when the phone rings, 'you get it, I don't want to talk to anybody.' This continues on-going and comes to the point requests may be made to lie, like 'I'm asleep, taking a bath and such.' Also, then you hear the 'I don't care' attitude for things that may need attention. In hindsight, this is obviously when she was losing her ability to talk in sentences and she was fully aware of it before we were. She was too embarrassed to talk to her friends on the phone, knowing she could not fully communicate with them and they would notice. This is also a period of inactivity except the usual, like laundry, basic meal preparation, and limited house work. A lot of hours are spent lying on the couch, taking naps. This is also a period of argumentative state that is triggered with merely a question, a statement, or an act of doing something different from the norm. This change is highly charged and requires kid gloves to diffuse. Most all visits with friends and family are greatly reduced with this stage.

In Faye's situation, mental attitude follows the physical attitude whereby simple things she had been able to perform now become difficult, aggravating, embarrassing, and downright refusal to perform in some cases. Case in point, balancing the checkbook has become too complicated and difficult to do. On a couple occasions she forgot to put the water in the coffee pot while making coffee, her inability to complete a thought when speaking at times. Often gets aggravated trying to set the VCR or set the clocks on the microwave and stove.

This is also a period of exaggeration whereby things are told with a slanted attitude that it is worse than it really is. In addition, some things are added to the real situation to make it sound worse. Pain now becomes severe at times but when in the company of others, it doesn't seem to be hardly present at all. The physical attitude worsens to the point that now she is unable to get out much at all other than for doctors appointments. No more grocery shopping or travel to anywhere that is not necessary. The ability to ride around in the car for an hour in the city is okay but travel to a destination that is an hour away is out of the question. Sarcastic and hateful verbal responses continue on an increase but only in private, seldom if ever in the presence of others.

It seems like Faye is now having irritable bowel syndrome. This was originally thought to be caused by the surgical removal of the gall bladder years ago, since there was often diarrhea seemingly on a scheduled basis. Like when the fluid has no where to go but to be absorbed, it appeared to build up and was then released in the form of diarrhea. This, of course, is not a scientific or professional opinion, but my own. Then, there is the problem of reflux, GERD, and prescribed medication to curb. One was Prevacid, ultimately prescribed and suddenly bowel urges became too quickly to get to the bathroom. This is one of the problems with this medication, so that medication is changed to another, Prilosec, with the understanding it would not be as bad. It seemed to cause the same problems. So, both were discontinued but apparently this has proven not to be the case and in the next few months or so there have been numerous 'accidents' in the bed, in the hallway, in the kitchen, and in the bathroom, too late. This has, therefore, halted all vacation travel and limited all shopping and visits to friends and family.

Next in line of noticeable changes was reduced strength. Faye now has trouble getting in and out of the bathtub, opening medicine bottles, and other tasks previously not a problem. This has been especially true in getting out of the bathtub. Three straight times in a week she was not able to get out and on one occasion suffered a fall back into the tub, bumping her upper back and head against the tile wall and tub. Needless to say, no more tub baths without assistance getting out or resort to showers instead. Then she started falling. First, she slid off the bed onto the floor. Then there was a fall or slide off the sofa chair onto the floor. A few days later she fell in the hallway gathering clothes to be laundered. Each case she required assistance in getting up and appeared dazed. There was no warning, no injuries, and no memory of what caused the falls.

The IBS accidents slowed to very infrequent but Faye's decision making and stammering increased. Words do not come easy in conversation, as if the thought process leaves, and often unable to finish a sentence. Two outings in the previous two weeks she had difficulty in ordering dinner either from words not flowing or indecision on what to order. A change in arthritis medicine seemed to help the leg pain but we wonder if this has caused confusion over taking another medication for another problem thinking this change also affects that medication which it does not. The new medication was for bursitis in the left leg below the knee and arthritis in right hip which was causing pain in the right thigh down to the right knee. This problem dramatically showed an increase in visible and verbal complaints of pain in both legs. Her appetite, or lack thereof, now was getting to be a problem. All she wants for lunch is cheese and crackers.

We noticed she was unable to recognize the value of money when she had her hair cut. The cost is $9.00 plus she usually gives the lady $2.00 for gratuity. On this occasion she gave the girl a $10.00 tip for the $9.00 haircut. When I questioned it she said didn't have any $1.00 bills. The lady also thought this was out of line and said no to the $10.00 but would accept $5.00 instead. We agreed to avoid any further embarrassment.

In mid May 2006 we discussed the problems with our family doctor during her regular checkup and he referred her to a psychiatrist for memory testing. He also schedule an MRI for her to try to determine whether the hip or back was causing the thigh pains which had become more intense since she had an epidural injection that had shown no improvement.

The pain in the thigh area became so severe and after two trips to the emergency room it was finally diagnosed that most likely the hip was causing the pain and we proceeded with our orthopedic surgeon to do total right hip replacement. Evidently this was the problem, not the back and not the knees. Most all of the pain was gone after six weeks recovery for the hip operation.

More blood work was scheduled. A carotid scan came back negative and not the source for her memory condition. The tests that were performed by the psychiatrist were done in two sessions with a third session for review. His diagnosis was bottom line global brain lapse rather than specific parts of the brain which resulted, obviously, in a very low score. Two possibilities he told us were: 1. lack of oxygen during surgery, 2. possible trauma from surgery which possibly could have aroused a problem that could have been in dormancy possibly for several years. A stroke would have affected the area only where stroke occurred and not global. Therefore, borders on Alzheimer's dementia was the conclusion. His recommendation was follow up with a neurologist.

Faye was still trying to help me do the cooking, cleaning, laundry, and whatever, best she could. One incident she put dry flour in hot frying pan for cube steak instead of rolling the steak in the flour first. Another incident she put dry corn meal in hot frying pan for cornbread instead of mixing it into a batter first. She urinated in the bathroom wastebasket and it slid out from under her causing her to fall flat on the floor in the puddle of urine in the middle of the night. After preparing a sandwich, she spread mayonnaise on the outside of the bread instead of butter to toast it, with the butter dish sitting right next to the sandwich. Her ability to make conversation continued to be a problem as if certain words don't come and it becomes a problem for me to decipher what is being said, sometimes she gets agitated. She now refused to talk to anyone on the telephone but if she answers the phone while I am outside and I ask who called she doesn't know. I had to ask her not to answer the phone at any time and let the answering machine pick it up.

Her neurologist visit results were the MRI image appears the brain is shrinking and in conjunction with the psychiatrist analysis, Faye's problem was consistent with Alzheimer's. He followed this with a brain wave test for further analysis and prescribed Aricept 5mg once daily and she continues taking this medication today. In the meantime the IBS problem increased like she has no idea when her bowels move until after the fact. The additional blood tests and the brain wave scan found no sign of blood vessel restrictions to the brain, bringing him back to his original diagnosis of Alzheimer's. According to her family doctor records, Faye had now lost approximately 70 pounds since her first knee replacement surgery which was December 1999, about six years earlier. I recently read that the rapid weight loss of a person not necessarily obese but overweight has been identified as another signal for dementia. Faye was weighing about 190-200 pounds which was somewhat overweight, but she was what we called a big bone person. So, this may be proof that this assumption may be correct.

The neurologist tried to add Namenda to the Aricept, but it apparently was too strong for Faye. It appeared to make her something between dizzy and nauseated so Namenda was discontinued but she continued taking Aricept.

I noticed her ability to recognize money was now completely gone. I asked her to get me 16 cents out of the car console where we keep loose change when getting ice cream and she handed me two quarters. I repeated 16 cents and she added two nickels. I then asked specifically for one nickel, one dime and one penny and she couldn't tell the difference.

Faye is now in her third year since diagnosed with Alzheimer's in 2006 and, frankly, I can't tell if she is getting any worse at all most days. Others it is obvious but she definitely hasn't gotten any better. She is responsive to commands from the physical therapist working with her but sometimes needs repeating and actually showing what procedure is being requested If in fact it is Alzheimer's/dementia, even if it was caused by loss of oxygen or extreme trauma, I think the Aricept is helping in the slowing of further deterioration. However, the incontinent problem is constant now. Seldom does she let me know in time. She still is unable to speak in conversation but can repeat any word you ask her to. We communicate like playing charade games. She needs assistance in her medication, bathing, dressing, and mobility. She adequately feeds herself and can point to what she wants on a menu at a restaurant but can't say it. We eat out a lot to keep her active outside the house and invite the boys and their families about once a week to a nice restaurant. Otherwise, I do what is required to maintain our household environment and I will take care of her as long as it is physically possible.

Now in our mid-seventies, it's a long way from Owl Hill but we have certainly enjoyed the journey and all the good times and you would think the 55 years together could never be taken away from us but think again, it can.

Faye remembers none of it.

Chapter 20

BONUS POEM SELECTIONS

From: *FIFTY YEARS OF LOVE POEMS*

By: Harold Hinson

This is a sampling of my collection of poems that I have written over the years. The working title of this collection is, appropriately enough, *FIFTY YEARS OF LOVE POEMS.* I hope you enjoy them.

LOVE STORM

The midnight air, pale moon above,
A perfect scene for the art of love.
The sounds of the sea just nearby,
The birds still singing their last cry.

The city lights so far away,
From the peaks that nearby lay.
Seem to utter their own song,
In rhythm as they flicker on.

And as the breeze across the hill,
Whispers gently, a sudden chill,
Seems to find its way through,
To make loves warmth feels so true.

Then the mighty clouds form around,
And lightning shines across the ground.
The mighty thunder loud and hard,
Then the rain splashed across the yard.

And as the rain ceased once more,
The love is cold, almost a bore.
The seas not angry, the city sleeps
The love is gone, but memories weep.

CANDLE OF LOVE

This is the story of a fellow in love,
In love with a lass, a gift from above.
Young in their heart and in their years,
So young indeed, could bring many tears.

Their love was so strong, it even glowed,
In their eyes and actions it showed.
They were happy and proud and yet,
They didn't know how rough it would get.

Time was slowly creeping them by,
Only a few times had brought a cry.
And then it happened one sad day,
That he would have to go far away.

The love that bound tightly back home,
Lingered on softly and on and on.
But time was working day and night,
To dowse the flame and cut the light.

The fight was on and in the end,
The flame flickered but returned again.
Never once did it fail to shine,
Into the heart of fate and time.

Reunion came once more to those,
That loved and shared their gift of woes.
That were conquered and all left behind,
To continue the love so young and kind.

FEELING OF SYMPATHY

There is so little one can say,
When sorrow comes in its cruel way.
And there is so little one can do,
No matter how much they really want to.

Words can't begin to help in need,
But feeling is truly a help indeed.
My feelings for you at a time like this,
Reaches deep inside with heavenly bliss.

He may have been a wonderful man,
I'm sure he was and in God's plan.
We have to learn to love and live,
And bear the fate our Lord will give.

He will help us through all our trials,
He will always follow our miles,
Wherever we travel, far or near,
These words, they are for you dear.

SECRET ADMIRATION

Though I have traveled far and near,
Never did I see a Miss so dear.
So gentle and kind and happily,
Enjoying life as it is, remarkably.

With a personality of her very own,
Distinctive taste, and so very grown.
Small she is and long is her hair,
That reveals so very delicate care.

She adores herself that I must say,
By observing her in a modest way.
For I have yet known her for real,
Cause she is only a dream I feel.

The girls I've known I won't discuss,
Have always been more I than us.
Until my eyes met her that time,
My heart fluttered and lost its rhyme.

I admire her so much indeed,
I write these words to relieve the need.
Because she exist in my mind,
Yet I doubt my path, she'll ever find.

THE LONGEST WAIT

The tenderness of love we had,
Made contact, we were so glad.
The longest wait had just begun,
Now nature had to make its run.

Old Father Time just laughed and said,
It won't be long, and scratched his head.
And he was right, up to the end,
But then, the longest wait began.

I walked the floor continuously,
To find relief and sympathy.
Thoughts of love and kindness too,
A simple prayer to help us through.

The hours passed, slowly by,
I waited for that lonesome cry.
I wished that I could ease the pain,
But, this I knew was in vain.

At last the time was drawing near,
I knew I had to be right here.
To share the gift of God above,
To cherish and eternally love.

My eyes grew heavy and very weak,
My body felt almost a heap.
And then, the longest wait no more,
Our baby came, from God's own door.

Loneliness is Fear

Have you ever been lonely, have you been afraid.
Or have you even wondered the difference it made.
Think of when you were lonely, think way back hard.
Think where you were so lonely, was it in the yard.

Or was it in the movie, how about the dream.
Or were you thinking of her, your best girl I mean.
You wonder if she's alright, or is she not well.
Or if she is even at home, just can't ever tell.

You wonder if she loves you, is she really true.
Or is she just an old tramp, just living off you.
You think she is happy, you think she is true.
It is you that is unhappy, because you are blue.

You are scared of everything, even a fast move.
Not many things can cure it, not even a sooth.
There's no soothing will do it, but don't shed a tear.
Here is the trouble darling, loneliness is fear.

When the loneliness is gone, the fear goes along.
Don't ever say you're lonely, the fear is not gone.
Tell her you love her often, and hold your head high.
I never will be lonely, fears will pass me by.

Move that lonesome feeling out, tell it to yourself.
You're not really that lonely, not small like an elf.
Think it over when you've time, but don't shed a tear.
'Cause if you do get lonely, loneliness is fear.

GODS TREES

So many words have been said
About the trees above our head.
So great they are, reaching high,
Up toward the beautiful cloudless sky.

The leaves sprouting out in spring,
From twigs and limbs for us bring,
Shade and comfort from the sun,
As well as beauty for everyone.

And the mighty trunk of a tree,
When cut and hewn gracefully,
Makes our homes greatest décor,
With all its beauty door to door.

And standing close to a tree so tall,
We are then so very, very small.
We feel that it has conquered us,
But yet, we're still courageous.

'Cause we know the tree has no mind,
To rule or teach things of any kind.
But, if it were not for the tree,
Our lives would only be helplessly.

THE LITTLE THINGS

One look into your beautiful eyes,
I see the beauty there that lies.
Just waiting for that special one,
To take to you to his world alone.

A tender kiss from your sweet lips,
Creates a splendor of exotic trips,
That never ends or pulls away,
Until nature has her own way.

The soft touch of your lovely skin,
Tends to light a fire within,
That burns with tender loving care,
For someone with a true desire.

And a perfect smile for every day,
To greet the world regardless what may,
Accepting daily ups and downs,
With active leaps, jumps and bounds.

And though much pain has been before,
The greatest effort has closed the door,
To most of life's unhappy rings,
Happiness comes from, the little things.

THE WICKED ONE

Is there such a love beyond compare,
In this cruel world of self desire.
That in itself, is truth and care,
Of one's own self without despair.

Can ones' love become a sudden sin,
And leave the heart saddened within,
With no escape for such a plight,
With no hope to win the lonely fight.

Can one be loved by only one,
Rather than two, should it be none.
Or will it be the sin of love,
That we have two gifts from above.

Who can be sure of himself, alone,
That love is here or love is gone.
How can we as only humans on,
This earth, determine, the wicked one.

OH MOTHER DEAR

Oh mother dear, why did you leave me?
Oh mother dear, why did you go away?
Oh mother dear, I love you truly,
Please tell me why, it was this way.

There once was a woman that was so near,
She was a mother, she was so dear,
She was the one that gave me birth.
She was the one sweetest thing on earth.

She was the one that loved and cared,
She was the one with her love shared.
She was the one through thick and thin,
Lived her life with a smile and grin.

She was the one that tucked me in,
Read to me and warned me of sin.
She was the one each and every day,
Stayed on my mind happy and gay.

Then one day so unexpectedly,
She became an angel and memory.
A memory of love and devotional care,
That only a mother could ever share.

OUR GIFT OF FIVE

How could one be so undermine,
To take for granted these things so fine.
The things that God has given us,
To use until we return to dust.

Our eyes were made for us to see,
The work of art or what it may be.
Placed on earth to each one of us,
To see and to know how wondrous.

And our hands were made for us to feel,
These things to believe if they are real.
And shape and mold what we touch,
Into the forms which we love so much.

Then we hear the remarkable song,
Of movement and joy moving along.
And never stop to understand,
That we're hearing in this promise land.

And as we wander here and there,
We smell the freshness of the air.
We smell the flowers all in bloom,
And watch them grow to perish soon.

And at the close of a beautiful day,
We hunger for food on our tray.
The taste so good fills our need
Yet these things are for granted indeed.

SOUTHERN STYLE

Now way down South in tobacco land,
Below Virginia but above the sand,
You'll find the place we love to stay,
North Carolina, I'm proud to say.

Tobacco is the leader in line,
But corn and beans right behind,
'Taters' and wheat and everything good,
Trees, which make the best of wood.

Watermelons, plums, peaches and pears,
Animals, all kinds, including bears,
You'll find the best in everything,
In North Carolina, in winter or spring.

Horseback riding, boating too,
Hunting deer, rabbits, foxes too.
Golf or skate, this is the place,
North Carolina simply holds the ace.

If you don't believe what I'm telling you,
Where else can you get all this to do,
Without the smog, smoke and jam,
Here's like Heaven, home of country ham.

ACKNOWLEDGEMENTS

The events described in this book are true to the best of my knowledge. What I have shared is what I know, what I saw, what I heard, or what I was told. Some names have been changed to protect the innocent but all places named are actual places. Special thanks go to my two sons, Todd and Scott (I always refer to them in order of their birth), for their willing and continued support and their computer knowledge when I need it. I also give special thanks to Derrick Hinson, my nephew, for his historical input with the Gentry family ancestors. And, most of all, thanks to my wife, Faye, for the many, many years of love and happy days we have spent together.

Made in the USA
Middletown, DE
29 August 2024

59969419R00092